ICD-11 IN AMERICA

A CLINICAL GUIDE TO THE FUTURE OF DIAGNOSIS

ELIZABETH M TEKLINSKI

INTEGRAL NEUROSCIENCE INITIATIVE

CONTENTS

ICD-11 IN AMERICA

A Clinical Guide to the Future of Diagnosis

Foundations, Clinical Domains, and Preparation for U.S. Adoption

INTEGRAL NEUROSCIENCE INITIATIVE

Elizabeth Teklinski, PhD, LPC, NCC, NPT-C

Michelle O'Connor-Teklinski, LMSW

Andrew Teklinski, MD, MS, FACC, CCDS, RPVI

ICD-11 in America: A Clinical Guide to the Future of Diagnosis

ISBN: 979-8-9942581-2-5

First Edition

Published by Integral Neuroscience Initiative
Traverse City, Michigan
www.integralneuroscience.org

For the clinicians who see beyond the code
to the patient beneath.

FOREWORD

The International Classification of Diseases represents one of the most sustained collaborative achievements in modern medicine. For over a century, the World Health Organization and its predecessor organizations have worked to create a shared language for describing human illness. This language enables clinicians to communicate across borders, researchers to aggregate findings across populations, and health systems to plan services based on comparable data. ICD-11, adopted by the World Health Assembly in 2019 and implemented globally since 2022, represents the most significant revision of this language in a generation.

What is often missed in discussions of classification is that these changes are not abstract. They determine whether certain conditions can be named at all, whether populations can be counted, and whether research findings can be compared across systems. When a condition lacks a coherent diagnostic home, patients experience the consequences long before policymakers do. ICD-11 emerged not only from scientific advance, but from decades of accumulated clinical friction.

The development of ICD-11 drew on contributions from thousands of clinicians, researchers, and public health experts across nearly every country in the world. It reflects advances in our understanding of disease mechanisms, incorporates conditions that previous editions could not adequately capture, and introduces structural innovations that allow for unprecedented diagnostic precision. The chronic pain classification, the approach to neurodevelopmental conditions, the dimensional model for personality disorders, and the recognition of post-viral syndromes all represent responses to clinical realities that previous systems addressed poorly or not at all.

Yet the existence of a global standard does not guarantee its adoption, and adoption does not guarantee understanding. Each country must translate the international classification into its own regulatory, administrative, and clinical context. This translation is neither automatic nor trivial. It requires attention to local health system structures, payment mechanisms, workforce preparation, and the practical realities of clinical documentation. Countries that have moved furthest in ICD-11 implementation have invested substantially in education, training, and systems adaptation.

The United States occupies a particular position in this global transition. American researchers and clinicians contributed significantly to the development of ICD-11, and American institutions remain deeply engaged with the World Health Organization on classification matters. At the same time, the complexity of the U.S. healthcare system, with its multiple payers, regulatory bodies, and deeply embedded administrative processes, creates implementation challenges that differ in kind from those faced by countries with more centralized health systems. The transition from ICD-9 to ICD-10 in the United States required coordination across federal agencies, private payers, software vendors, and hundreds of thousands of healthcare providers over more than two decades. The eventual transition to ICD-11 will require similar coordination.

In this context, the need for guidance tailored to U.S. clinicians and health systems is evident. Most existing ICD-11 resources are designed for international audiences, focused on technical implementation details, or written for specialists in health information management. What has been lacking is a comprehensive resource that addresses the conceptual, clinical, and practical dimensions of ICD-11 from the perspective of American healthcare professionals who will eventually work within this system—and from an organization dedicated to bridging the gap between classification systems and clinical implementation.

This book fills that gap. It approaches ICD-11 not as a coding manual or policy document, but as a clinical and scientific framework that deserves careful understanding. The authors bring the perspective of practicing clinicians who have worked across multiple domains of healthcare, from mental health to chronic pain management to cardiovascular medicine. This breadth of experience informs an approach grounded in clinical reality rather than administrative abstraction.

What distinguishes this work is its tone and orientation. It does not press for immediate action or manufacture urgency. It does not advocate for particular policy positions or timelines. Instead, it offers explanation, context, and preparation. It treats readers as professionals capable of forming their own judgments when provided with accurate information. It respects the complexity of the U.S. healthcare system while maintaining clarity about what ICD-11 represents and why it matters.

The book moves systematically through the foundations of ICD-11, the clinical domains where changes are most significant, the research and data implications of improved classification, and the practical realities of preparation for eventual transition. Throughout, it maintains the measured perspective appropriate to a reference work intended for long-term use. Clinicians, researchers, health system leaders, and educators will find material relevant to their particular concerns, presented without the distortion that accompanies either resistance to change or enthusiasm detached from practical constraints.

Diagnostic classification evolves because medicine evolves. The conditions we recognize, the mechanisms we understand, and the distinctions we find clinically meaningful change over time. A classification system that served well in one era may constrain clinical thinking and research progress in the next. ICD-11 represents an effort to align diagnostic language with contemporary medical knowledge. Eventual U.S. adoption will bring American healthcare into alignment with the global standard that already governs mortality reporting and international health data exchange.

The timing and process of that alignment remain to be determined by the institutions responsible for such decisions. What clinicians can do now is prepare, and preparation begins with understanding. This book provides that understanding in a form accessible to those whose primary concern is patient care rather than classification theory or health policy. It is a valuable contribution to the literature on diagnostic classification. More importantly, it provides a foundation for informed engagement with a system that will increasingly shape clinical care, research, and health data in the years ahead.

Andrew H. Teklinski, MD, MS, FACC, CCDS, RPVI
Chief Medical Officer
Integral Neuroscience Initiative

PREFACE

Diagnosis is the foundation of clinical work. It shapes treatment decisions, determines access to services, organizes research, and structures communication among providers. When clinicians document a diagnosis, they are not simply selecting a code for administrative purposes. They are using a shared language to describe human suffering and to position that suffering within a framework that guides care.

This is why classification systems matter more than most clinicians realize. The categories available to us shape what we see, what we name, and ultimately what we do. When a condition lacks a code, it becomes invisible to research, to policy, and often to payers. When a code exists but misrepresents the clinical reality, patients carry a label that distorts their experience and may misdirect their care. The architecture of classification is never neutral.

When a diagnostic system fails to represent a condition accurately, the consequences are not theoretical. Patients struggle to access care for conditions their providers cannot name. Clinicians document what the system permits rather than what they observe. Researchers cannot study what cannot be reliably identified. Over time, these failures accumulate into systemic blind spots that persist for decades. ICD-11 is an attempt to correct some of those blind spots.

This book exists because the World Health Organization released a fundamentally revised classification system in 2019, and the United States has not yet adopted it. ICD-11 represents the first major revision to international disease classification in thirty years. It reflects advances in clinical science, addresses long-standing diagnostic gaps, and introduces structural innovations that ICD-10 could not accommodate. Over one hundred countries have begun implementation. The United States continues to operate on the previous system, creating a widening gap between American clinical practice and global standards.

This gap is not a failure of will or awareness. It reflects the complexity of American healthcare infrastructure, the scale of required coordination, and the competing demands on system modernization. The transition from ICD-9 to ICD-10 took twenty-five years after the WHO released the new system, involved multiple Congressional delays, and required massive investments across the healthcare ecosystem. Those who experienced that transition remember the disruption and remain cautious about repeating it prematurely.

ICD-11 differs substantially from its predecessor. The structural changes are significant. The clinical improvements are meaningful. And the timeline for American adoption, while uncertain, is not indefinite. The question facing clinicians today is not whether ICD-11 will arrive, but whether they will understand it when it does.

This book was written to prepare American clinicians for that moment. Most existing ICD-11 resources are designed for international audiences, written for technical specialists, or focused on specific clinical domains. What has been missing is a comprehensive guide that respects the U.S. context, addresses the concerns of practicing clinicians, and presents ICD-11 as what it is: a clinical and scientific evolution, not merely a bureaucratic change.

The chapters that follow move from conceptual foundations through specific clinical domains to practical preparation. They address chronic pain, autism and neurodevelopmental conditions, mental and behavioral health, and post-viral syndromes—areas where ICD-11 offers substantial improvements. They examine the U.S. context honestly and provide guidance for those who want to prepare before mandates create urgency.

This is not a coding manual. It will not make you a certified coder, nor does it attempt to replace the technical resources that coders and health information professionals require. Instead, it offers what I believe clinicians need first: conceptual understanding. Before anyone can use ICD-11 effectively, they must understand why it was built, how it differs from what came before, and what it makes possible that was previously constrained. That conceptual foundation is what this book provides.

This book will clarify how ICD-11 works, what its innovations mean for clinical practice, and how clinicians can begin preparing for transition. It will respect the complexity of the U.S. healthcare system and avoid pretending that adoption is simpler than it is. It will provide enough detail to support informed decision-making without overwhelming readers with technical minutiae.

What it will not do is advocate for immediate adoption, prescribe billing practices, or dictate clinical decisions. ICD-11 is a classification system, not a treatment protocol. The codes describe conditions; they do not determine what care is appropriate. That judgment remains where it belongs, with clinicians who know their patients. This book supports that judgment by improving diagnostic literacy. It does not substitute for it.

I am aware that many clinicians approach classification systems with ambivalence. Diagnosis can feel reductive, administrative, even dehumanizing when it fails to capture the complexity of individual patients. The ICD-10 transition was disruptive and costly. Skepticism about whether ICD-11 will improve anything meaningful is reasonable.

I share some of that skepticism. Classification systems are tools, not truths. They organize clinical reality in ways that are sometimes useful and sometimes distorting. No system perfectly captures the heterogeneity of human suffering. The question is not whether ICD-11 is perfect, because it is not. The question is whether it represents an improvement over what we have now, and in many domains the answer is clearly yes.

Consider chronic pain. For decades, clinicians treating patients with persistent pain conditions have worked within a diagnostic framework that was never designed for them. ICD-10 scatters pain codes across multiple chapters, reflects an outdated dualism between physical and psychological pain, and lacks categories for conditions that millions of patients experience. ICD-11 creates a dedicated chronic pain chapter built on contemporary pain science, distinguishes between primary and secondary pain in ways that align with clinical reality, and allows documentation of severity, functional impact, and psychological distress. This is not a minor administrative adjustment. It is a reconceptualization that validates patient experience and supports appropriate care.

Similar improvements appear throughout the system. The autism spectrum is now recognized as a unified condition with specifiers for intellectual development and functional language, resolving diagnostic inconsistencies that have affected service access for years. Post-viral syndromes have a place in ICD-11, relevant for the millions affected by Long COVID and other infection-associated chronic conditions. The personality disorder classification moves from rigid categories to a dimensional model that better captures clinical reality. These are not theoretical gains. They address problems that practicing clinicians encounter daily.

I have written this book for readers who take diagnosis seriously as clinical work. That includes physicians across specialties, mental health professionals, allied health providers, and the health system leaders, researchers, and educators who support clinical practice. It includes those who are curious about ICD-11 and those who are skeptical of it. It includes early adopters and cautious observers. All are welcome here.

What I ask of readers is openness. ICD-11 represents genuine advances in how medicine conceptualizes certain conditions. Understanding those advances requires setting aside assumptions formed by years of working within ICD-10. This does not mean accepting everything uncritically. It means engaging with the material as clinicians rather than as defenders of the status quo. The classification system will change eventually. The only question is whether you will understand what is changing when it does.

Preparation does not require urgency, but it does reward foresight. The timeline for U.S. adoption remains uncertain, yet the system that will eventually govern diagnosis documentation, research reporting, and health statistics has already been defined. Clinicians who invest in understanding now will find the eventual transition far less disorienting than those who encounter ICD-11 for the first time when compliance becomes mandatory. They will be better positioned to care for their patients, contribute to research, and lead their organizations through change.

This book is an invitation to begin.

Elizabeth Teklinski, PhD, LPC, NCC, NPT-C
Founder and President
Integral Neuroscience Initiative

INTRODUCTION

Every clinical encounter begins with a question: What is happening to this patient? The answer to that question, however provisional, sets everything else in motion. It determines what tests are ordered, what treatments are considered, what specialists are consulted, what the patient is told. Diagnosis is not a formality that follows clinical work. It is the cognitive act that organizes clinical work from the first moment of contact.

This understanding of diagnosis as clinical cognition is essential to everything that follows in this book. Diagnosis is not primarily about codes, although codes are how diagnoses are recorded and transmitted. It is not primarily about billing, although billing systems depend on diagnostic documentation. Diagnosis is how medicine makes sense of suffering. It is the translation of patient experience into categories that allow for reasoning, communication, and action.

The categories themselves come from classification systems. These systems are the invisible infrastructure of medicine, shaping clinical attention in ways that most practitioners never consciously consider. When a classification system includes a condition, that condition becomes visible to research, to epidemiology, to policy, and to payment. When a classification system excludes a condition, or represents it poorly, patients with that condition become harder to study, harder to count, and often harder to treat appropriately.

Classification systems do not merely record what medicine already knows. They structure what medicine can know. A researcher studying a condition that lacks a coherent diagnostic code faces immediate obstacles: no way to identify cases consistently across datasets, no way to aggregate findings across institutions, no way to compare prevalence across populations or time. The absence of a code is not a neutral gap. It is an active constraint on knowledge production.

When diagnostic language fails to reflect clinical reality, the consequences propagate quietly but pervasively. Conditions become difficult to study, services become difficult to justify, and patients encounter systems that cannot fully recognize what they are experiencing. Over time, these misalignments harden into structural blind spots that shape care long after their origins are forgotten. Classification reform is one of the few levers medicine has to address these blind spots at scale.

The same logic applies to clinical care. When diagnostic categories reflect the conditions clinicians actually encounter, documentation becomes an act of precision. When categories are outdated, overly broad, or conceptually confused, documentation becomes an act of approximation. Clinicians select the code that comes closest, knowing it does not quite fit. The resulting data misrepresents clinical reality, and decisions based on that data inherit its distortions.

This is the context in which classification systems must be understood. They are not administrative conveniences imposed on clinical work from outside. They are the conceptual scaffolding within which clinical work takes place. When the scaffolding is well designed, it supports accurate documentation, meaningful research, and coherent communication. When the scaffolding is poorly designed, it creates friction, introduces error, and constrains what medicine can accomplish.

The challenge is that classification systems age. Medical knowledge advances, clinical populations change, and conditions that once seemed rare or marginal become central concerns. A classification system designed for one era may become a constraint in the next. Categories that made sense when they were created may no longer align with how clinicians think, how researchers investigate, or how patients experience their conditions.

Classification is always provisional, representing the best available synthesis of knowledge at a given moment. The question is not whether a system will become outdated—it will—but how medicine responds when it does.

The International Classification of Diseases has been revised periodically since its origins in the late nineteenth century, each revision reflecting the accumulated advances of the intervening decades. ICD-11 is the latest in this sequence, incorporating thirty years of progress in understanding disease mechanisms, recognizing conditions that earlier systems could not adequately represent, and introducing structural features that allow for greater precision and flexibility.

The specific changes matter, and this book will examine them in detail. But before attending to specifics, it is worth pausing on the general principle: diagnostic classification is not static, and clinicians who understand the logic of classification are better positioned to use any system well. The goal of this book is not merely to explain what ICD-11 contains. It is to develop the kind of diagnostic literacy that allows clinicians to think clearly about classification itself.

This orientation shapes how the book approaches its subject. Rather than presenting ICD-11 as a set of rules to be memorized, it presents the system as an expression of clinical and scientific reasoning. Each major change reflects a substantive judgment about how a domain of medicine is best organized. Understanding those judgments requires understanding the clinical realities they address.

Chronic pain, for example, has never fit comfortably within classification systems designed around acute injury and organ-specific pathology. The changes in ICD-11 represent an attempt to bring classification into alignment with contemporary pain science, which recognizes chronic pain as a condition in its own right rather than merely a symptom of something else. Understanding this change requires understanding both the clinical problem it addresses and the scientific framework it reflects.

The same principle applies throughout the system. Neurodevelopmental conditions, mental and behavioral health, post-viral syndromes, and other domains all receive attention in ICD-11 because earlier classification frameworks did not adequately serve the clinicians and patients who work within them. In each case, understanding the change means understanding what was inadequate before and what the new approach makes possible.

This book is written for readers who want that deeper understanding. It assumes that clinicians are capable of engaging with the reasoning behind classification, not merely following instructions. It assumes that understanding precedes effective implementation, and that clinicians who grasp the logic of a system will use it more skillfully than those who learn it mechanically. It assumes, in short, that diagnosis is intellectual work deserving of intellectual engagement.

The timing of U.S. adoption remains uncertain, and this book does not depend on any particular timeline. What it offers is the opportunity to develop conceptual readiness now, while there is time to learn thoughtfully rather than reactively. Clinicians who understand ICD-11 before mandates arrive will be prepared to use it well. They will also be prepared to evaluate it critically, to identify where it succeeds and where it falls short, and to contribute to its ongoing refinement.

Classification systems are human creations, subject to revision and improvement. The clinicians who engage most deeply with any system are those best positioned to shape its future development. Understanding is not passive acceptance; it is the foundation for informed participation. With that foundation established, the next chapter examines ICD-11 as a global clinical language: how it functions, how it differs from prior systems, and why understanding its design is essential before considering its implications for American practice.

HOW TO USE THIS GUIDE

This book is designed as a reference work. It does not assume or require sequential reading. Readers may begin with the chapters most relevant to their professional context and return to other sections as needed. The structure supports both sustained reading and selective consultation.

Structure of the Book

The book is organized into four parts. Part I establishes the foundations of ICD-11, including the rationale for the revision, the key differences from ICD-10, the experiences of other countries in implementation, and the architectural features that distinguish the new system. Readers unfamiliar with ICD-11 may find it useful to begin here, though those with prior exposure may proceed directly to later sections.

Part II addresses clinical domains where ICD-11 introduces significant changes. These chapters examine chronic pain, autism and neurodevelopmental conditions, post-viral syndromes, and mental and behavioral health. Each chapter can be read independently. Clinicians working primarily in one domain may consult the relevant chapter without requiring material from other sections.

Part III examines the broader context of classification, including implications for research, epidemiology, and health data systems, as well as the current status of U.S. adoption efforts. These chapters are particularly relevant for those concerned with population health, quality measurement, or institutional planning.

Part IV focuses on practical preparation, addressing what clinicians and health systems can do now to build readiness for eventual transition. The final chapters discuss documentation practices, administrative considerations, and the relationship between classification and reimbursement. The appendices provide supplementary tools, including crosswalks, glossaries, and documentation templates.

Suggested Reading Paths

Different readers will approach this book with different purposes. Clinicians new to ICD-11 may begin with Part I, then turn to their relevant clinical domain. Those focused on specific conditions can read Part II chapters independently. Researchers and data specialists will find Part III most immediately useful. Health system leaders may begin with Parts III and IV. Educators can treat individual chapters as modular resources.

What This Book Does Not Require

This book does not prescribe adoption timelines, advocate policy positions, or require changes to current practice. It is not a coding manual or billing guide; readers needing technical coding resources should consult official guidelines. Nothing here replaces clinical judgment—diagnostic classification provides a framework for documentation, but interpretation and treatment decisions remain the clinician's responsibility. This book aims to improve diagnostic literacy, and readers may engage with it at their own pace.

Using the Book Over Time

This book is designed to remain useful over an extended period. As ICD-11 implementation progresses and U.S. adoption timelines become clearer, readers may return to relevant sections with new questions. The foundational material in Parts I and II will retain its relevance regardless of policy developments, while Parts III and IV address considerations that will become increasingly practical as transition approaches.

The appendices are intended as working tools. The crosswalks, glossary, and documentation templates may be consulted repeatedly as readers encounter specific classification questions in their practice or research. These resources complement the narrative chapters and can be used independently.

A Note on Preparation

Preparation for significant infrastructure change is gradual. This book provides the conceptual foundation on which practical skills can later be built. Readers who invest time in understanding now will find themselves better prepared when implementation timelines are established. Understanding precedes fluency, and this book provides the first step.

PART I

FOUNDATIONS

1

ICD-11 AS A GLOBAL CLINICAL LANGUAGE

Diagnosis is how medicine thinks. Before treatment begins, before prognosis is discussed, before a patient can be enrolled in a clinical trial or counted in an epidemiological study, there must be a diagnosis. The words clinicians use to name what is wrong with a patient shape everything that follows: what questions are asked, what tests are ordered, what treatments are offered, and how outcomes are measured. Diagnosis is not merely documentation. It is, as Feinstein (1967) observed, the organizing principle of clinical reasoning.

The International Classification of Diseases provides the vocabulary for this essential work. The World Health Organization defines this role explicitly:

The International Classification of Diseases (ICD) is the foundation for the identification of health trends and statistics globally, and the international standard for reporting diseases and health conditions. ICD provides a common language that allows health professionals to share health information across the world. (World Health Organization, 2019a)

For more than a century, the ICD has served as this global standard for recording diagnoses, tracking mortality, and comparing health data across populations. The system traces its origins to nineteenth-century efforts to standardize mortality statistics, building on foundational work by Farr (1839) and Bertillon (1903), with early advocacy from Florence Nightingale (1859) for uniform hospital statistics (Moriyama et al., 2011; Fagot-Largeault, 2006). In the United States, clinicians encounter this system every day, whether or not they realize it. Every diagnosis code entered into an electronic health record, every claim submitted to an insurer, every patient counted in a registry draws on ICD's structure and logic. The classification is so embedded in clinical infrastructure that most clinicians take it for granted, noticing it only when a code is difficult to locate or an insurance claim is denied.

Yet the version of ICD that American clinicians use is no longer the global standard. In May 2019, the Seventy-Second World Health Assembly adopted ICD-11 as the successor to ICD-10 (World Health Organization, 2019b). Implementation took effect globally in January 2022 (World Health Organization, 2022). By the time this sentence is read, most of the world will have moved on from the system the United States continues to use. This book explains what ICD-11 is, why it matters, and what American clinicians need to understand as the transition approaches.

Classification as Clinical Language

Classification systems are often discussed as though they were purely administrative instruments, relevant mainly to billing and compliance. This framing misses something fundamental. As Bowker and Star (1999) demonstrated in their influential study of classification systems, the categories we use to organize information shape what we can see and what we can know. Diagnosis is never neutral; it reflects cultural, scientific, and institutional contexts that evolve over time (Rosenberg & Golden, 1992; Jutel, 2011). A diagnostic classification is not merely a list of codes. It is a clinical language that determines which distinctions can be made, which patterns can be recognized, and which questions can be asked.

Consider what happens when a classification lacks a code for a condition that clinicians recognize in practice. Patients with that condition are either assigned a code that does not accurately describe their situation or relegated to an unspecified category that conveys almost nothing. Either way, the clinical reality disappears from the data. It cannot be tracked, studied, or counted. It cannot inform policy or guide resource allocation. For research purposes, it effectively does not exist.

This is not a theoretical concern. For years, clinicians working with patients who experienced prolonged symptoms after acute infections had no adequate diagnostic language. Codes for fatigue, for cognitive complaints, for autonomic dysfunction existed separately, but no classification recognized the constellation of symptoms as a coherent entity. Patients were coded according to their most prominent symptom, scattering what might have been a recognizable population across dozens of unrelated categories. The emergence of Long COVID brought sudden attention to this gap (Nalbandian et al., 2021), but the underlying problem predated the pandemic by decades (Komaroff & Bateman, 2021).

Similar limitations appear throughout clinical medicine. Chronic pain, complex trauma, and autism spectrum conditions have all been inadequately served by classification systems that could not capture their clinical reality. In each case, the limitation was not primarily bureaucratic. It was conceptual. The classification lacked the language to describe what clinicians observed.

ICD-11 represents a systematic effort to address these limitations. Harrison et al. (2021) describe the scope of this effort:

ICD-11 is no longer a static list of disease names. It is built on a semantic knowledge base, referred to as the Foundation, which contains all ICD entities and their relationships. From this Foundation, linearizations can be derived for specific uses, including mortality and morbidity statistics. (Harrison et al., 2021, p. 206)

The development of ICD-11 involved rethinking the architecture of classification rather than simply adding new codes to an existing structure. Over 300 specialists from 55 countries participated in working groups, with input from thousands of clinicians and researchers worldwide (World Health Organization, 2019c). The goal was not merely to update code values but to modernize the conceptual foundations of diagnostic classification itself.

Table 1.1. ICD Version Comparison

FEATURE	ICD-10	ICD-11
Release Year	1990	2019
Architecture	Static hierarchical list	Foundation + linearizations
Total Entities	~14,000 codes	~85,000 entities
Update Cycle	Multi-decade revisions	Annual updates
Post-coordination	Not supported	Extension codes
Chronic Pain	Scattered across chapters	Dedicated chapter
Digital Design	Print-based origin	Digital-native

The Structural Limits of ICD-10

The World Health Organization released ICD-10 in 1990. At that time, the Human Genome Project had just begun, HIV treatment remained rudimentary, and electronic health records existed only in experimental form. The scientific understanding of many conditions has transformed since then. Pain science has moved from purely biomedical models to recognition of central sensitization and nociplastic mechanisms (Kosek et al., 2021; Fitzcharles et al., 2021). Autism research has established the condition as a neurodevelopmental difference rather than a behavioral disorder (Lord et al., 2018). Trauma studies have documented the distinct presentations of prolonged and repeated trauma (Brewin et al., 2017). Mental health research has increasingly questioned categorical diagnoses in favor of dimensional and transdiagnostic approaches (Kotov et al., 2017).

ICD-10 cannot capture these advances. Its structure predates them. Clinicians working with chronic pain patients, for instance, find themselves navigating a scattered landscape of codes distributed across multiple chapters with no unifying framework. Treede et al. (2019) articulate the clinical significance:

Chronic pain is defined as pain that persists or recurs for longer than three months. In some conditions, such as fibromyalgia or nonspecific low back pain, chronic pain may be conceived as a disease in its own right rather than a symptom of another condition. In the ICD-11 classification, these conditions are grouped under the term chronic primary pain. (Treede et al., 2019, p. 20)

Pain is coded in ICD-10 primarily by anatomical location rather than mechanism, forcing clinicians to choose between imprecise options that do not reflect contemporary understanding of pain conditions. A patient with fibromyalgia receives one code; the same patient's chronic headache receives another; neither code indicates that both symptoms may reflect a common underlying process of central sensitization (Fitzcharles et al., 2021).

The problem extends beyond specific clinical domains. ICD-10's architecture is categorical in a rigid sense. Patients either meet criteria for a diagnosis or they do not. Severity, functional impact, and symptom dimensions must be inferred from code selection rather than documented explicitly. Comorbidity is captured through multiple codes, but the relationships between conditions cannot be expressed within the classification itself.

For research, these limitations create significant barriers. Cohort identification depends on the precision of diagnostic codes. When codes are imprecise, heterogeneous populations are grouped together, obscuring treatment effects and confounding outcome analysis. Epidemiological studies struggle to compare data across institutions and countries when the same code may be applied with different clinical interpretations (Jetté et al., 2010). These are not complaints about administrative burden. They are observations about the constraints that an outdated classification system places on clinical thinking, clinical communication, and clinical research.

The Architecture of ICD-11

ICD-11 was designed to address these limitations through architectural innovation rather than incremental revision. The World Health Organization describes the foundational change:

ICD-11 has been developed to be fit for the digital age. It is the first classification to be entirely electronic in its production, and it is designed to be used in digital health environments. The Foundation component of ICD-11 contains all the content of the classification in a form that is amenable to scientific analysis and digital manipulation. (World Health Organization, 2022, ICD-11 Reference Guide)

The most significant structural change is invisible to casual users but essential to understanding how the system works. ICD-11 is built on a foundation layer containing the complete ontology of all classified entities, approximately 85,000 in total. This foundation is not itself a coding system. It is the knowledge base from which coding systems are derived.

Different linearizations, or subsets of the foundation organized for specific purposes, serve different users. The primary version most clinicians will encounter, ICD-11 for Mortality and Morbidity Statistics (MMS), contains approximately 17,000 diagnostic categories (Harrison et al., 2021). This architecture allows the classification to be maintained continuously as medical knowledge evolves. The WHO now releases annual updates, incorporating new evidence and correcting errors without requiring another multi-decade revision cycle.

Beyond architecture, ICD-11 introduces post-coordination: the capacity to combine a primary diagnosis with extension codes that add detail about severity, anatomy, temporality, etiology, and other dimensions. Rather than requiring a unique pre-coordinated code for every possible clinical scenario, which would result in millions of codes, ICD-11 allows clinicians to build precise descriptions from a manageable set of components.

The diagnosis becomes a structured clinical description rather than a label selected from a limited menu. Chapter 4 examines this architecture in detail, including the Foundation, linearizations, and the mechanics of post-coordination.

ICD-11 also introduces dimensional thinking in specific clinical domains. Reed et al. (2019) describe the changes in mental and behavioral health classification:

The ICD-11 approach to the classification of mental disorders represents a major shift from previous practice. The classification is organized based on a developmental lifespan approach, and dimensional elements have been added to what has traditionally been a categorical classification. (Reed et al., 2019, p. 4)

The personality disorder classification, for example, replaces categorical types with a severity-based model that captures mild, moderate, and severe presentations along with trait domain qualifiers (Bach & First, 2018; Tyrer et al., 2015). This allows clinicians to describe the degree and character of personality pathology rather than selecting from predefined categories that may not fit individual patients.

Similar innovations appear throughout the classification. Chronic pain receives its own chapter with mechanism-based categories (Treede et al., 2019). Autism spectrum disorder is classified with specifiers for intellectual functioning and language capacity, allowing dimensional description of a condition long recognized as heterogeneous (Greaves-Lord et al., 2022). Complex PTSD is recognized as distinct from single-incident trauma. Brewin (2020) describes the distinction:

Complex PTSD is characterized by the core symptoms of PTSD together with disturbances in self-organization, including affect dysregulation, negative self-concept, and disturbances in relationships. These additional features are associated with prolonged or repeated traumatic events from which escape is difficult or impossible. (Brewin, 2020, p. 146)

These changes represent responses to clinical realities that prior classification systems addressed inadequately. In each case, the revision reflects accumulated evidence and clinical consensus rather than administrative convenience.

The United States in Global Context

The United States has not adopted ICD-11. At the time of this writing, there is no federal mandate, no official implementation timeline, and no U.S. clinical modification in development. American clinicians continue to use ICD-10-CM, a system the WHO retired years ago.

This situation reflects structural features of the U.S. healthcare system rather than ideological resistance. The fragmented infrastructure of multiple payers, thousands of independent health systems, and complex regulatory coordination means any classification change propagates through billions of annual claims.

The ICD-10 transition illustrates the challenge: the WHO released ICD-10 in 1990, but the United States did not implement ICD-10-CM until 2015 (Topaz et al., 2013). That experience—with multiple postponements, compressed preparation, and significant transitional costs—shaped institutional caution about the next change. Chapter 10 examines the U.S. adoption landscape in detail.

None of this means that ICD-11 adoption will not occur. The United States has adopted every prior revision of the ICD eventually. The question is not whether but when, and under what conditions. Meanwhile, global health research increasingly uses ICD-11 terminology. International clinical guidelines reference ICD-11 categories. Multinational research collaborations require ICD-11 literacy for participation.

Jakob and Dee (2021), writing in the WHO Bulletin, describe the global implementation landscape:

ICD-11 implementation is progressing across all WHO regions. Early adopters have demonstrated that implementation is feasible when supported by adequate preparation, training, and stakeholder engagement. Countries that invested in education and systems adaptation have reported smoother transitions than those that treated implementation as primarily a technical exercise. (Jakob & Dee, 2021, p. 204)

American clinicians face a practical challenge. They work within a system that has not officially adopted ICD-11, yet the conceptual and scientific advances embedded in ICD-11 are relevant to clinical practice regardless of coding requirements. Understanding ICD-11 is not merely preparation for an eventual regulatory mandate. It is engagement with the contemporary state of diagnostic classification science.

Scope and Boundaries of This Book

This book is a clinical guide, not a coding manual. It is designed to help American clinicians understand ICD-11 conceptually, anticipate the transition practically, and apply ICD-11's advances in their clinical thinking today. It is not a comprehensive code reference. It is not a billing guide. It does not predict regulatory timelines or advocate for specific policy positions.

The chapters that follow build understanding progressively, from foundational concepts through specific clinical domains to practical preparation.

Throughout, the emphasis is on conceptual understanding rather than technical detail. Code values and classification hierarchies change. Underlying concepts are more durable. A clinician who understands why ICD-11 introduced mechanism-based pain classification will be prepared to use that classification effectively whenever it becomes available. The same clinician who merely memorizes code numbers will need to start over when codes change.

The reality is that ICD-11 already matters, regardless of U.S. adoption status. It matters for research literacy, as international studies increasingly use ICD-11 terminology. It matters for clinical thinking, as ICD-11's conceptual advances reflect the current scientific understanding of many conditions. It matters for preparation, as organizations that begin building awareness now will face less disruption when formal transition requirements eventually arrive.

Understanding as Foundation

The language clinicians use to describe their patients shapes what they can see and what they can communicate. A classification system that cannot name a condition makes that condition invisible to systems that depend on classification data. A system that fragments a coherent syndrome across unrelated categories prevents recognition of patterns that might inform treatment. A system that forces categorical choices where dimensions would be more accurate distorts clinical communication.

ICD-11 represents an effort to bring diagnostic classification closer to clinical reality. Its dimensional elements, its mechanism-based categories, its capacity for post-coordinated description, and its recognition of conditions long overlooked by prior classifications all serve clinical purposes. These are not administrative conveniences. They are tools for clinical thinking.

Madden and Musgrove (2020) articulate the broader vision:

ICD-11 offers the potential for a more powerful health information system, one that is flexible enough for future modification and capable of supporting the increasingly complex demands of clinical care, research, and public health. Realizing this potential will require sustained investment in education, implementation, and ongoing maintenance. (Madden & Musgrove, 2020, p. 5926)

American clinicians did not choose to be left behind in this transition. The delay reflects systemic factors beyond any individual's control. But clinicians can choose how they respond to the situation. They can wait passively for mandates, scrambling to comply when deadlines arrive. Or they can begin learning now, building expertise and organizational readiness that will serve them regardless of when official adoption occurs.

The chapters that follow build on this foundation. Chapter 2 examines the structural limitations of ICD-10 and the specific problems that ICD-11 was designed to solve.

2

THE LIMITS OF ICD-10

The International Classification of Diseases has been revised periodically since its origins in the late nineteenth century. Each revision reflects the accumulated medical knowledge of the intervening decades, incorporating new conditions, refining existing categories, and responding to the evolving needs of clinicians, researchers, and public health authorities. ICD-10, released by the World Health Organization in 1990, represented a substantial expansion over its predecessor, increasing the number of available codes and introducing greater specificity in many clinical domains. For three decades, it has served as the global standard for mortality and morbidity statistics.

Yet the world in which ICD-10 was designed no longer exists. The Human Genome Project had not yet produced results. The internet was not yet a feature of clinical practice. Electronic health records were experimental curiosities rather than regulatory requirements. The scientific understanding of many conditions has transformed in the intervening years. Pain science, trauma psychology, autism research, and infectious disease epidemiology have all advanced in ways that ICD-10 could not have anticipated and cannot adequately represent.

Understanding ICD-11 requires understanding what necessitated it. The eleventh revision is not merely an updated code list. It represents a fundamental reconceptualization of how diagnostic classification systems should be built and maintained. The changes address both the content limitations of ICD-10, the conditions it represents poorly or not at all, and the structural limitations that prevented the system from evolving as medical knowledge advanced.

The Structural Constraints of ICD-10

ICD-10 was designed in the late 1980s, finalized before the widespread adoption of digital health systems. Its structure reflects this origin. The classification exists as a hierarchical list of codes with associated inclusion and exclusion terms, organized into chapters by body system or condition type. This architecture served well for paper-based coding and statistical tabulation. It does not serve well for the demands of contemporary health informatics.

Harrison et al. (2021), in their comprehensive overview of ICD-11, describe the fundamental problem:

While ICD-10 has long been used in digital forms, properties that reflect its pre-digital origin constrain tooling and data exchange, impede maintenance and development, and have enabled differences of structure and meaning to creep into translations and modifications. (Harrison et al., 2021, p. 2)

This observation captures several distinct problems. First, ICD-10's structure constrains the tools that can be built around it. The classification lacks the semantic richness needed for sophisticated decision support, natural language processing, or automated coding assistance. Second, the structure impedes maintenance. Changes to ICD-10 require careful attention to cascading effects across the hierarchy, and structural characteristics limit the types of modifications that can be made without disrupting existing uses. Third, and perhaps most consequentially, the structure has allowed divergence across implementations. Different countries, different clinical modifications, and different translations have introduced variations in meaning that undermine the comparability the classification was designed to ensure.

The authors elaborate on the accumulating pressure for revision:

Since the development of ICD-10, medicine has advanced, and the understanding of many diseases has changed substantially. The modifications needed to accommodate these changes exceeded what could be achieved by simply updating the 10th revision. (Harrison et al., 2021, p. 2)

This is a crucial point. The WHO did attempt to update ICD-10 through an established mechanism for incorporating new knowledge. However, structural characteristics of the classification and requirements for continuity limited what changes could be made. A growing list of desired modifications accumulated, deferred for the eventual eleventh revision. The problem was not merely that specific codes were missing or outdated. The problem was architectural: the system's design prevented it from evolving at the pace of medical knowledge.

Consider the practical consequences. A researcher seeking to study chronic primary pain conditions could not identify a coherent cohort using ICD-10 codes, because the classification scattered relevant codes across multiple chapters with no unifying framework. A clinician documenting a patient with complex PTSD had no code that captured the condition's distinctive features. A health system attempting to track post-viral syndromes found that patients with similar presentations received different codes depending on which symptoms predominated, making epidemiological analysis impossible. These are not marginal concerns. They represent systematic failures of the classification to serve its intended purposes.

Table 2.1 summarizes the key structural limitations of ICD-10 and their clinical consequences.

Table 2.1. ICD-10 Structural Limitations

LIMITATION	ICD-10 CONSTRAINT	CLINICAL CONSEQUENCE
Rigid Architecture	Static hierarchical list; major revisions require decades	Classification falls behind advancing medical knowledge
Categorical Rigidity	Fixed categories without dimensional specifiers	Severity and function cannot be captured systematically
Chapter Fragmentation	Related conditions scattered across multiple chapters	Chronic pain, sleep disorders lack coherent representation
No Post-coordination	Single codes only; no mechanism for combining concepts	Complex presentations require approximation or multiple codes
Pre-digital Origin	Designed for paper; digitized retrospectively	Limited integration with EHR and decision support systems
Semantic Limits	No formal ontology; limited machine-readability	Poor interoperability; translation divergence across systems

The Need for Architectural Redesign

The decision to undertake a major revision of the ICD reflected recognition that incremental updates could not address the accumulated limitations. What was needed was not a larger code list but a different kind of classification system entirely. Harrison et al. (2021) identify the fundamental shift:

Changes in content reflect knowledge and perspectives on diseases and their causes that have emerged since ICD-10 was developed about 30 years ago. Changes in design and structure reflect the arrival of the networked digital era, for which ICD-11 has been prepared. (Harrison et al., 2021, p. 1)

This distinction between content changes and structural changes is essential. Content changes, adding new codes, refining existing categories, reorganizing chapters, could in principle be accomplished within ICD-10's existing architecture, albeit with difficulty. Structural changes required starting from different foundational assumptions about what a classification system should be and how it should work.

The structural redesign addressed several related objectives. The new system needed to support multiple use cases without requiring separate, potentially divergent modifications. It needed to accommodate continuous updating as medical knowledge evolved. It needed to integrate with digital health information systems rather than merely being digitized after the fact. And it needed to maintain semantic consistency across translations and implementations.

These objectives led to the most significant innovation in ICD-11: the separation of the underlying knowledge base from the classifications derived from it. Rather than creating a single hierarchical code list, as in previous revisions, the developers created a comprehensive ontology of medical concepts from which multiple fit-for-purpose classifications could be generated.

The Foundation and Derived Classifications

ICD-11's architecture differs fundamentally from all previous revisions. Harrison et al. (2021) describe the core innovation:

ICD-11's information framework comprises a semantic knowledge base (the Foundation), a biomedical ontology linked to the Foundation and classifications derived from the Foundation. ICD-11 for Mortality and Morbidity Statistics (ICD-11-MMS) is the primary derived classification and the main successor to ICD-10. (Harrison et al., 2021, p. 1)

The Foundation is the comprehensive repository of all ICD entities: diseases, disorders, injuries, external causes, signs and symptoms, and extension entities. It contains approximately 85,000 distinct clinical concepts, each defined with standardized properties including definitions, synonyms, inclusion and exclusion terms, and relationships to other entities. The Foundation is not itself a coding system. It is the knowledge base from which coding systems are derived.

This architecture enables several capabilities that were impossible under ICD-10. Different linearizations, organized subsets of the Foundation for specific purposes, can serve different users without requiring separate maintenance efforts. The primary linearization, ICD-11 for Mortality and Morbidity Statistics (ICD-11-MMS), contains approximately 17,000 diagnostic categories and is the direct successor to ICD-10 for most clinical and statistical purposes. Other linearizations serve specialized needs: primary care, dermatology, mental health, and other domains can have tailored versions that draw from the same underlying knowledge base.

The separation of Foundation from linearization also enables continuous maintenance. When medical knowledge advances or errors are identified, changes can be made to the Foundation and propagated to derived classifications in a controlled manner. The WHO now releases annual updates to ICD-11, incorporating new evidence without requiring the multi-decade revision cycles that characterized previous transitions. This is not merely convenient. It means the classification can remain current with medical science rather than falling progressively further behind.

Digital-Native Design

Perhaps the most consequential difference between ICD-11 and its predecessors is that ICD-11 was designed from the outset for digital environments. This represents a fundamental shift informed by decades of research on controlled medical vocabularies. Cimino (1998) articulated key desiderata for such systems, including concept permanence, unique identifiers, and formal definitions—principles now embedded in ICD-11's architecture. Harrison et al. (2021) emphasize this point:

Fundamental to making the ICD fit for the digital age has been to base it on a computable knowledge framework. This is the most important difference between ICD-11 and earlier revisions. Introduction of a knowledge framework has enabled ICD-11 to be interoperable in digital health information environments. (Harrison et al., 2021, p. 3)

The implications of this design choice extend throughout the system. Each entity in the Foundation has a unique, permanent identifier that remains stable even as the entity's name or classification position changes. This enables reliable data linkage across time and systems. The semantic structure of the Foundation supports automated reasoning, allowing software to infer relationships and validate coding choices. ICD-11's architecture also facilitates mapping to other major terminologies, including SNOMED CT (Rodrigues et al., 2015) and integration with the Unified Medical Language System (Bodenreider, 2004). The architecture supports application programming interfaces (APIs) that enable remote access to ICD-11 content and services, integrating the classification directly into electronic health record systems and other digital tools.

The authors note that while ICD-11 can still be used in paper-based systems, the advantages of electronic use are substantial:

Though ICD-11 can be used in paper-based systems, the tools and capabilities made possible by the framework are expected to make electronic use compelling for most users. (Harrison et al., 2021, p. 3)

The online coding tool exemplifies this digital-native approach. Unlike the alphabetical index that accompanied previous ICD versions, the ICD-11 coding tool provides intelligent search functionality, suggests relevant extension codes, validates postcoordinated combinations, and offers guidance on code selection. Field testing indicates that this approach produces more consistent and accurate coding than traditional methods (Harrison et al., 2021).

Postcoordination and Extension Codes

One of the most significant practical innovations in ICD-11 is postcoordination: the ability to combine a primary diagnosis code with extension codes that add clinically relevant detail. This addresses a fundamental tension in classification design. A precoordinated system, in which every possible clinical scenario has its own unique code, would require millions of codes and become unusable. A purely postcoordinated system, in which clinicians build diagnoses from atomic components, would sacrifice the standardization that makes classification valuable.

ICD-11 adopts a hybrid approach. Stem codes represent the primary diagnostic concepts, comparable in scope to ICD-10 codes. Extension codes, contained in a dedicated supplementary chapter, capture additional dimensions: severity, laterality, temporality, anatomy, etiology, and other clinically relevant characteristics. Clinicians can combine stem codes with appropriate extension codes to create precise diagnostic descriptions without requiring a unique precoordinated code for every permutation.

The extension code chapter contains codes for concepts including disease stage, severity scales, histopathology, anatomical detail, and diagnosis timing. When linked to a stem code, these extensions allow multidimensional coding that captures clinical complexity far beyond what ICD-10 permitted. A diagnosis of moderate chronic low back pain with significant functional limitation, for example, can be expressed precisely rather than approximated by selecting the closest available code from a limited menu.

Postcoordination is supported by sanctioning rules embedded in the coding tool. These rules specify which combinations are permitted, preventing clinically nonsensical or redundant code clusters. The system guides users toward appropriate combinations while maintaining the flexibility to capture clinical nuance. This represents a significant advance over ICD-10, where clinicians often had to choose between precision and standardization.

Content Innovations

The architectural changes in ICD-11 enabled substantial content innovations that would have been difficult or impossible under the previous structure. Several new chapters address clinical domains that lacked coherent representation in ICD-10.

Chapter 7, Sleep-Wake Disorders, consolidates conditions previously scattered across multiple chapters, reflecting the maturation of sleep medicine as a distinct clinical discipline. Chapter 17, Conditions Related to Sexual Health, provides a framework for conditions that were awkwardly placed or inadequately represented in earlier classifications. Chapter 21 organizes symptoms, signs, and clinical findings in a more clinically useful structure.

Most significantly for many clinicians, ICD-11 introduces a dedicated chapter for chronic pain. Chapter MG30 organizes chronic pain conditions according to contemporary pain science, distinguishing chronic primary pain, where pain is the condition itself, from chronic secondary pain, where pain accompanies another diagnosed condition. This reflects decades of research demonstrating that chronic pain involves distinct mechanisms and requires distinct clinical approaches regardless of original etiology.

Mental and behavioral health classification also received substantial revision. The dimensional approach to personality disorders replaces rigid categorical types with a severity-based model that better captures clinical reality. Complex PTSD is recognized as distinct from single-incident trauma. Autism spectrum disorder is unified with specifiers for intellectual functioning and language capacity. Gaming disorder and compulsive sexual behavior disorder receive recognition as diagnosable conditions.

These content changes were informed by extensive consultation with clinical experts, professional societies, and patient advocacy groups. Working groups for each clinical domain reviewed evidence, proposed revisions, and conducted field testing to assess the utility and reliability of proposed categories. The result is a classification more closely aligned with contemporary clinical practice than any previous ICD revision.

Implications for Transition

The scope of changes between ICD-10 and ICD-11 has implications for how transition will proceed. Unlike the transition from ICD-9 to ICD-10, which primarily involved learning a new code structure and expanded code set, the transition to ICD-11 involves conceptual changes in how diagnosis is represented and communicated.

Clinicians will need to understand not just new codes but new capabilities: postcoordination, extension codes, the distinction between Foundation and linearization, and the logic underlying reorganized chapters. Health information systems will need to accommodate code clusters rather than single codes, implement postcoordination tools, and integrate with ICD-11's digital infrastructure. Administrative processes built around ICD-10's structure will require adaptation.

At the same time, the WHO designed ICD-11 with transition in mind. A design objective was to maintain reasonable backwards comparability with ICD-10, particularly for important conditions. The overall chapter structure remains similar, and many high-level categories map directly between versions. Detailed mapping tables support data continuity across the transition period.

The architectural innovations that distinguish ICD-11 from previous revisions also offer advantages for transition. The continuous update mechanism means that issues identified during implementation can be addressed promptly rather than accumulated for a future revision. The digital tools built into ICD-11 can guide users through coding decisions, reducing the learning burden. The Foundation's comprehensive concept definitions support training and education.

Understanding the design principles behind ICD-11 provides context for the specific clinical changes examined in subsequent chapters. The chronic pain classification, the autism spectrum reconceptualization, the recognition of complex PTSD, and the accommodation of post-viral syndromes all represent applications of the architectural principles described here. In each case, the new classification captures clinical reality that ICD-10 could not represent, enabled by structural innovations that made such representation possible.

3

GLOBAL ADOPTION

The World Health Assembly adopted ICD-11 in May 2019. Implementation became effective for member states on January 1, 2022. These facts establish that ICD-11 is now the official global standard for disease classification. What they do not reveal is the considerable variation in how countries have approached adoption, the different stages at which national health systems currently operate, and the practical realities that have shaped implementation decisions across diverse healthcare contexts.

This chapter examines global adoption of ICD-11 as it has actually occurred rather than as policy documents might suggest it should occur. The picture that emerges is one of heterogeneity: different countries at different stages, pursuing different pathways, facing different constraints. Understanding this variation is essential context for American clinicians, who work within a system that has not yet begun formal transition but will eventually need to navigate the same territory.

Adoption as Process, Not Event

The transition from one classification system to another is not a single decision implemented on a fixed date. It is a process that unfolds over years, involving multiple stakeholders, substantial infrastructure changes, and iterative refinement of tools and training. The World Health Organization has consistently communicated this understanding to member states. The official WHO implementation guidance states explicitly:

Countries can continue to use ICD-10 for as long as necessary, but prompt adoption of ICD-11 is encouraged to ensure interoperability, consistency with global standards, benefit from ongoing enhancements, and compliance with international commitments. (World Health Organization, n.d.)

This language is notable for what it does and does not say. It encourages adoption without mandating a timeline. It acknowledges that countries face different circumstances. And it frames the benefits of transition in terms of data quality and global coordination rather than regulatory compliance or penalty avoidance.

The WHO has also been explicit that no penalties attach to delayed implementation:

There is no penalty for countries that do not meet the implementation timeline. WHO recognizes that each country may face unique technical, financial, or organizational challenges. Nonetheless, delaying implementation may impede the benefits of up-to-date medical classification and hamper global data comparability and interoperability. (World Health Organization, n.d.)

This framing matters because it establishes the context in which national decisions are made. Countries are not racing against a deadline with consequences for failure. They are making strategic choices about when and how to invest in classification infrastructure, balancing the benefits of modernization against the costs and disruptions of transition.

Current Global Status

As of late 2024, WHO reports indicate that 132 member states and areas are at various phases of implementing ICD-11. This figure represents substantial global engagement with the new classification. However, the distribution across implementation stages reveals the graduated nature of adoption.

Approximately 72 countries have commenced the implementation process, which includes translation efforts and initial planning activities. Another 50 countries are conducting or expanding implementation pilots, testing ICD-11 in specific settings or for specific use cases before broader deployment. Fourteen countries and areas have begun collecting or reporting data using ICD-11 coding for at least some purposes.

These figures illustrate that full implementation remains the exception rather than the rule even several years after ICD-11 became officially effective. Most countries engaged with ICD-11 are in preparatory or pilot phases. This pattern reflects the substantial work required to transition classification systems, particularly in countries with established ICD-10 infrastructure and complex health information ecosystems.

Table 3.1 provides an overview of adoption stages across selected countries, illustrating the variation in approach and progress.

Table 3.1. Global ICD-11 Adoption Status by Country

COUNTRY	SYSTEM TYPE	STAGE	CURRENT FOCUS
Kuwait	Centralized	Routine use	Mortality and morbidity coding
Saudi Arabia	Centralized	Gradual integration	Hospital system expansion
Germany	Decentralized	Preparation	Translation and tooling
Canada	Decentralized	Assessment	Roadmap development
Australia	Decentralized	Assessment	Cost-benefit analysis
United States	Decentralized	Pre-assessment	No official timeline

Note: Stages reflect status as of late 2024 and are subject to change. Health system characterizations are simplified for comparative purposes.

The adoption process itself follows recognizable patterns across countries, regardless of where they currently stand. Countries typically progress through sequential stages of increasing integration, from initial preparation through pilot testing to routine use.

Factors Shaping Adoption Pathways

The variation in adoption progress reflects systematic differences in how countries approach classification transitions. Several factors consistently influence the pace and character of implementation.

Health system centralization affects coordination requirements. Countries with unified national health systems can make implementation decisions at a single point and propagate them throughout the system. Countries with fragmented or federated health systems must coordinate across multiple independent actors, each with their own timelines, budgets, and priorities. The difference is not merely administrative. It shapes whether implementation can proceed as a coordinated national project or must emerge from the accumulated decisions of many independent organizations.

Existing ICD infrastructure creates path dependencies. Countries that have invested heavily in ICD-10 clinical modifications, associated coding workforces, and integrated billing systems face higher transition costs than countries using the WHO base version with less elaborate local adaptations. The United States, with ICD-10-CM containing over 70,000 diagnosis codes and deeply integrated into payment systems, represents an extreme case. Countries without clinical modifications face simpler transitions but may have less developed coding capacity to begin with.

The relationship between classification and payment systems matters substantially. In countries where diagnosis codes directly determine reimbursement through diagnosis-related groups or similar mechanisms, any classification change affects financial flows throughout the health system. The stakes of transition are correspondingly higher, and the tolerance for disruption lower. Countries that use ICD primarily for statistical purposes without tight payment linkages can pilot new systems with less immediate financial consequence.

Workforce considerations shape feasible timelines. Training coders to use a new classification system requires time and resources. Countries with well-established health information management professions can build on existing competencies. Countries with less developed coding workforces may find that ICD-11's integrated tooling reduces training requirements compared to ICD-10, but still face capacity constraints.

Patterns in Early Adoption

Examination of countries that have moved furthest toward ICD-11 implementation reveals several consistent patterns. These are not prescriptions but observations about what has characterized successful early progress.

Early adopters typically began with mortality coding rather than morbidity coding. Mortality statistics involve smaller data volumes, more standardized processes, and clearer international reporting requirements than the full range of clinical coding. Starting with mortality allows countries to develop institutional familiarity with ICD-11 in a relatively controlled context before addressing the more complex morbidity use case.

Pilot testing has been a consistent feature of successful transitions. Rather than attempting system-wide implementation at once, countries have typically selected specific hospitals, regions, or use cases for initial deployment. These pilots generate practical experience, identify unexpected challenges, and build the evidence base needed to plan broader implementation. The WHO explicitly supports this approach, providing guidance on pilot design and evaluation.

Dual coding periods, where cases are coded in both ICD-10 and ICD-11 simultaneously, have helped countries assess the practical implications of transition. Dual coding reveals where the new system captures information differently, where training gaps exist, and what adjustments to workflow or documentation may be needed. It also generates the mapping data necessary to maintain historical comparability across the transition.

Investment in training and tooling has preceded successful implementation. The WHO has emphasized that ICD-11's digital design reduces but does not eliminate training requirements. Countries that have progressed furthest have typically invested in developing local training capacity, translating materials into national languages, and adapting the WHO coding tools to local information systems.

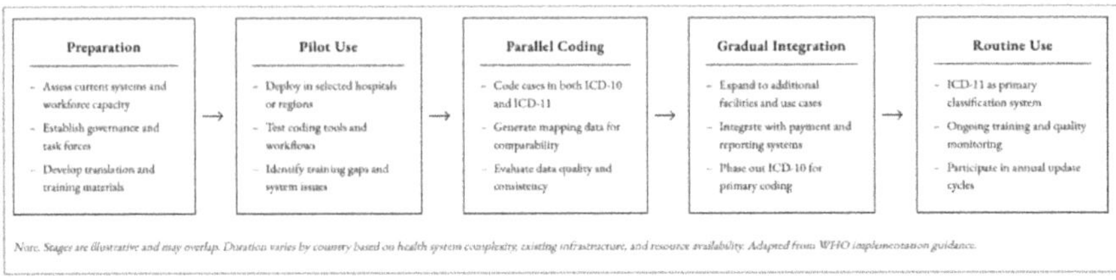

Figure 3.1. Typical ICD-11 Adoption Pathway

Lessons from Implementation Experience

Several years of global implementation experience have generated practical insights that inform how subsequent adopters approach transition. These lessons emerge from published accounts of pilot programs, WHO technical consultations, and the accumulated experience of early-adopting countries.

The WHO has synthesized key observations from early implementation:

Transitioning to ICD-11 is a collaborative and iterative process involving stakeholders from the clinical, administrative, research, and policy sectors. By staying informed, actively sharing updates, and embracing the global momentum, countries and organizations can ensure a smooth and timely transition that benefits patients, health systems, and global health surveillance efforts. (World Health Organization, n.d.)

This characterization as collaborative and iterative merits emphasis. Implementation has not proceeded as top-down mandates executed on fixed schedules. It has involved ongoing dialogue between those who develop classification systems and those who use them, with adjustments made in response to practical experience. The WHO's maintenance process for ICD-11, which allows for annual updates, supports this iterative approach in ways that were not possible with previous revisions.

Stakeholder engagement emerges as a consistent theme in successful implementations. Clinical input on whether new codes capture clinical reality, coding professional input on workflow implications, IT input on system integration, and administrative input on resource requirements all shape how implementation proceeds. Countries that engaged these stakeholders early report smoother transitions than those that treated implementation as primarily a technical exercise.

The importance of clear governance structures has become evident. Successful implementations typically involve designated lead agencies with authority to coordinate across institutional boundaries. National task forces or steering committees that bring together health ministries, statistical agencies, payer organizations, and professional bodies have helped align the many actors whose cooperation is necessary for system-wide transition.

Resource requirements have been significant but variable. The WHO estimates that a member state newly introducing ICD-11 in a simple information system may need one to two years, while states with highly sophisticated systems where earlier ICD versions are deeply embedded may require substantially longer. The variation in estimated timelines reflects the diversity of starting points and system complexity across countries.

Implications for Later Adopters

Countries that have not yet begun ICD-11 implementation can draw several conclusions from global experience to date. These conclusions inform the preparation strategies discussed in later chapters of this book.

First, delay is not unusual. Most countries with established ICD-10 infrastructure have not yet reached full ICD-11 implementation. The United States is not uniquely slow; it is part of a large cohort of countries still in early stages of transition planning. The complexity of American healthcare infrastructure makes transition particularly challenging, but the fact of delayed adoption is typical rather than exceptional.

Second, preparation time is valuable. Countries that have invested in understanding ICD-11 before formal implementation timelines were established report being better positioned when transition begins. This suggests that clinicians, health systems, and policymakers who engage with ICD-11 now, even absent regulatory mandates, will be better prepared than those who wait.

Third, the character of transition can be shaped by early decisions. Countries make choices about whether to adopt the WHO base version or develop clinical modifications, whether to transition mortality and morbidity coding simultaneously or sequentially, and how tightly to couple classification change with payment system reform. These choices have lasting consequences for implementation complexity and timeline.

Fourth, ICD-11's design accommodates gradual transition. Unlike previous revisions, ICD-11 was built with implementation realities in mind. The architecture supports multiple use cases from a common foundation. The digital tooling can be integrated into existing systems. The annual update process allows for refinement based on implementation experience. These design features make phased implementation more feasible than it was for previous classification transitions.

Global Adoption in Perspective

ICD-11 is real, operational, and in use globally. The classification is no longer a future prospect but a present reality, with data being collected and reported under ICD-11 codes in multiple countries. At the same time, full global adoption remains years away. Most countries, including most with sophisticated health information systems, are still in preparatory or pilot phases.

This heterogeneous picture has implications for how American clinicians should understand their situation. The United States has not been left behind by a world that has uniformly moved to ICD-11. Rather, it is part of a varied global landscape in which countries at different stages are finding their own pathways to adoption. The experience of early adopters provides lessons that can inform American preparation, but does not provide a single template to be copied.

What the global picture does establish is that ICD-11 works. It can be implemented. It generates usable data. It integrates with existing health information systems. The questions facing countries like the

United States are not whether ICD-11 is viable but when and how to undertake the transition. Those questions are addressed in subsequent chapters, beginning with a detailed examination of ICD-11's architecture and continuing through the specific clinical domains where the new classification offers the most significant advances.

4

THE ARCHITECTURE OF ICD-11

The previous chapters have established that ICD-11 exists, that it differs substantially from ICD-10, and that countries around the world are adopting it through varied pathways. What remains to be explained is how ICD-11 actually works. This is not a question about coding procedures or implementation logistics. It is a question about the fundamental structure that makes ICD-11 capable of representing clinical reality in ways that previous classification systems could not.

Understanding this architecture matters for clinicians, not just informaticians. The structural choices embedded in ICD-11 determine what can be expressed, what distinctions can be made, and what information can flow from clinical documentation into research, epidemiology, and health system management. A clinician who understands the architecture will recognize why certain coding options exist, why certain combinations are possible, and why the system behaves as it does. This understanding supports effective use of the classification regardless of which specific codes or categories apply to a given clinical domain.

This chapter explains ICD-11's architecture at a conceptual level. It describes what the Foundation is and why it matters, how linearizations derive from the Foundation, what post-coordination enables, and how extension codes expand the system's expressive capacity. The goal is comprehension, not technical mastery. Readers should finish this chapter understanding why ICD-11 had to be built the way it was built, not how to perform coding operations within it.

From Lists to Knowledge Structures

Previous versions of the ICD were fundamentally lists. They organized diseases and conditions into hierarchical categories, assigned codes to those categories, and provided inclusion and exclusion terms to guide classification decisions. This structure served well for statistical tabulation and mortality reporting. It did not serve well for the complex demands of contemporary clinical documentation, research data aggregation, or digital health information exchange.

The limitation was not merely that ICD-10 lacked certain codes. The limitation was architectural. A hierarchical list can only express what has been pre-defined within it. Every distinction that might be clinically relevant must have its own code, or it cannot be captured. As medical knowledge expanded and clinical documentation became more detailed, the number of potentially relevant distinctions grew far beyond what any manageable code list could accommodate.

ICD-11 addresses this constraint by reconceptualizing what a classification system should be. Rather than a list of codes, ICD-11 is built on a semantic knowledge base: a structured repository of clinical concepts and their relationships. Chute and Çelik (2022) describe the architectural transformation:

The architecture for ICD-11 proposed in 2007 included three layers: a semantic network of biomedical concepts (Foundation), a traditional tabulation of hierarchical codes that would derive from that network (Linearization), and a formal ontology that would anchor the meaning of terms in the semantic network. (Chute & Çelik, 2022, p. 2)

This three-layer architecture separates the comprehensive representation of clinical knowledge from the specific code structures used for particular purposes. The Foundation contains everything the classification knows about diseases and health conditions. Linearizations extract subsets of that knowledge organized for specific use cases. The ontological layer ensures that terms have consistent, computable meanings across all contexts.

Table 4.1. ICD-10 vs. ICD-11 Architecture Comparison

FEATURE	ICD-10	ICD-11
Entity representation	Single location per entity	Multiple parenting permitted
Expressiveness	Pre-coordinated codes only	Pre- and post-coordination
Clinical detail	Fixed by code definition	Extensible via modifiers
Use case adaptation	Country modifications	Derived linearizations
Update mechanism	Accumulated revisions	Annual Foundation updates

Note. The architectural shift from ICD-10 to ICD-11 enables greater flexibility, precision, and maintainability in diagnostic classification.

The ICD-11 Foundation

The Foundation is the comprehensive repository of all ICD-11 entities. It contains approximately 85,000 distinct clinical concepts, including diseases, disorders, injuries, external causes, signs, symptoms, and the extension codes discussed later in this chapter. Each entity in the Foundation has a unique identifier that remains stable regardless of how the entity is used in any particular classification context.

The Foundation differs from a traditional code list in several important respects. First, it permits multiple parenting. A condition can belong to more than one conceptual category simultaneously. Diabetic nephropathy, for example, is both an endocrine disorder and a kidney disease. In ICD-10, it must be placed in one chapter or the other, with cross-references indicating its relevance elsewhere. In the ICD-11 Foundation, it exists as a single entity with relationships to both domains, and linearizations can position it according to their specific purposes.

Second, the Foundation supports continuous maintenance. Changes to knowledge about diseases, including new conditions, refined definitions, and corrected relationships, can be incorporated into the Foundation without waiting for a full revision cycle. The WHO now releases annual updates to ICD-11, with changes propagating from Foundation to linearizations in a controlled manner.

Third, the Foundation provides semantic richness beyond what a code list can offer. Each entity carries standardized properties: textual definitions, synonyms and search terms, inclusion and exclusion criteria, and relationships to other entities. This structured information supports clinical decision tools, natural language processing, and automated coding assistance in ways that were impossible with previous ICD versions.

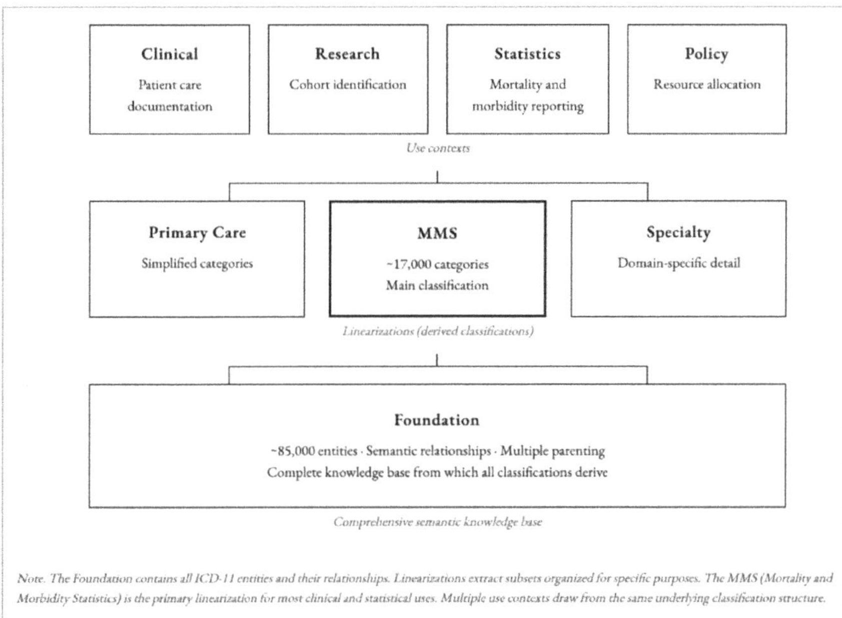

Figure 4.1. ICD-11 Code Structure. The Foundation contains all ICD-11 entities and their relationships. Linearizations extract subsets organized for specific purposes. The MMS (Mortality and Morbidity Statistics) is the primary linearization for most clinical and statistical uses. Multiple use contexts draw from the same underlying classification structure.

Linearizations: Purpose-Specific Classifications

The Foundation is not itself a coding system. It is the knowledge base from which coding systems are derived. Linearizations are those derived coding systems: organized subsets of Foundation content structured for specific use purposes. The primary linearization, ICD-11 for Mortality and Morbidity Statistics (MMS), contains approximately 17,000 diagnostic categories and serves as the direct successor to ICD-10 for most clinical and statistical applications.

The linearization concept addresses a practical problem that plagued previous ICD versions. Different users need different things from a classification system. A primary care provider needs broad, clinically intuitive categories. A specialist needs fine-grained distinctions within their domain. A researcher needs consistent, reliable categories for cohort identification. A health administrator needs categories that support resource planning and population health monitoring. A single code list cannot optimally serve all these purposes.

ICD-10 attempted to address this problem through national clinical modifications, with countries developing their own extended code sets. This approach created divergence: ICD-10-CM in the United States contains over 70,000 codes, while other countries use different modifications or the base WHO version. Cross-national comparison became complicated, and the proliferation of modifications made WHO maintenance more difficult.

ICD-11's linearization architecture offers an alternative. Rather than modifications layered on top of a base version, ICD-11 envisions multiple linearizations derived from the same Foundation. The MMS serves most general purposes. A primary care linearization can present simplified categories appropriate for that setting. Specialty linearizations can offer domain-specific detail. All draw from the same underlying knowledge base, maintaining conceptual alignment even as they differ in granularity and organization.

Post-Coordination: Building Precise Diagnoses

Perhaps the most significant practical innovation in ICD-11 is post-coordination: the ability to combine a primary diagnosis code with additional codes that specify clinically relevant details. This addresses a fundamental tension in classification design that constrained all previous ICD versions.

Consider the clinical scenario of a patient with moderate chronic low back pain causing significant functional limitation. In ICD-10, the clinician might code M54.5 (Low back pain), possibly adding G89.29 (Other chronic pain) to indicate chronicity. But the system provides no structured way to document that the pain is moderate in severity, that it significantly limits function, or that it represents a primary pain condition rather than pain secondary to another diagnosis. This information exists only in clinical notes, invisible to research and analytics.

A pre-coordinated system, where every possible clinical scenario has its own unique code, cannot solve this problem. The combinations of condition, severity, chronicity, laterality, etiology, and functional impact would require millions of codes. The system would become unusable, and even then would lack codes for combinations the developers did not anticipate.

ICD-11 adopts a hybrid approach. Stem codes represent primary diagnostic concepts, comparable in scope to ICD-10 codes. Extension codes, contained in a dedicated supplementary chapter, capture additional clinical dimensions. Clinicians combine stem codes with appropriate extension codes to create precise diagnostic expressions, called clusters, without requiring unique pre-coordinated codes for every permutation.

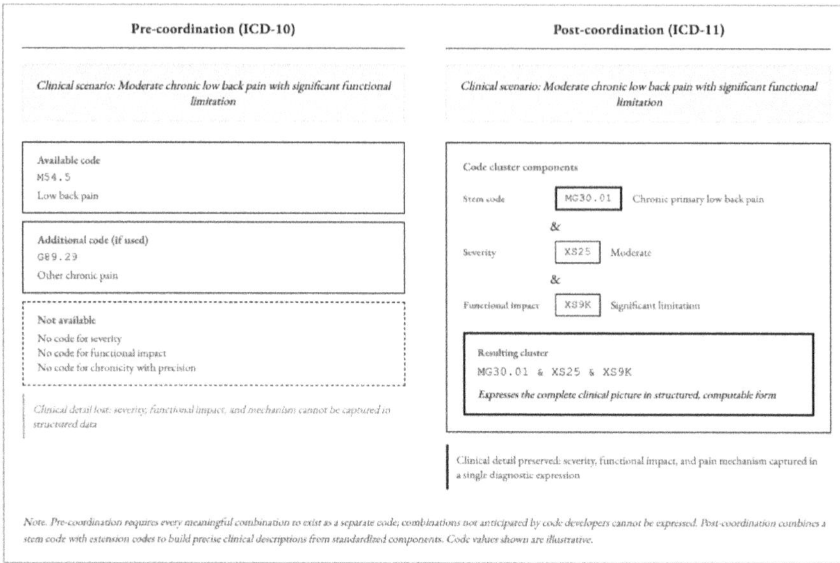

Figure 4.2. Pre-coordination versus Post-coordination. Pre-coordination (ICD-10) requires every meaningful combination to exist as a separate code; combinations not anticipated by code developers cannot be expressed. Post-coordination (ICD-11) combines a stem code with extension codes to build precise clinical descriptions from standardized components. Code values shown are illustrative.

Extension Codes and Clinical Dimensions

Extension codes are the building blocks of post-coordination. They occupy a dedicated chapter in ICD-11 (Chapter X), containing codes that cannot stand alone as diagnoses but add clinically relevant information when combined with stem codes. Understanding extension codes as dimensions of description rather than add-ons clarifies their function.

Severity codes allow documentation of how significantly a condition affects the patient. Rather than requiring separate codes for mild, moderate, and severe presentations of every condition, a single severity dimension can modify any condition for which severity is clinically meaningful. The coding system does not predetermine which conditions can have severity specified; that determination emerges from clinical judgment about what information matters for a given case.

Temporality codes capture the time course of conditions. Acute, subacute, chronic, and recurrent presentations can be distinguished. For conditions where the temporal pattern affects prognosis or treatment, this information becomes part of the diagnostic expression rather than being lost or relegated to free text.

Anatomy and laterality codes specify location. Laterality eliminates ambiguity for conditions affecting paired structures. Anatomical detail codes extend this principle to more specific localization within body regions, enabling precise documentation of where conditions manifest.

Etiology codes link conditions to their causes when those causes are known and clinically relevant. A secondary condition can be explicitly connected to the primary condition that produced it, maintaining the relationship in structured data rather than relying on code sequence or narrative documentation.

Functional impact codes, drawing on concepts from the International Classification of Functioning, Disability and Health (ICF), allow documentation of how conditions affect patients' capacity to perform activities and participate in life situations. This integration addresses a long-standing gap between disease classification and functional assessment.

Table 4.2. Extension Code Categories

CATEGORY	DESCRIPTION AND PURPOSE
Severity	Documents degree of clinical impact (mild, moderate, severe)
Temporality	Captures time course (acute, chronic, recurrent)
Anatomy	Specifies anatomical location and laterality
Etiology	Links conditions to causes; maintains causal relationships
Histopathology	Captures tissue-level findings for oncology and pathology
Functional Impact	Documents effects on activity and participation (ICF)
Diagnosis Timing	Indicates when diagnosis was made relative to encounter
Medication	Associates conditions with therapeutic agents
Healthcare Activity	Documents associated procedures and interventions

Note. *Extension codes cannot stand alone as diagnoses. They modify stem codes to create post-coordinated clusters. Sanctioning rules determine which combinations are permitted.*

Stem Codes and Cluster Codes

The distinction between stem codes and cluster codes is fundamental to understanding how ICD-11 expresses diagnoses. A stem code represents a primary diagnostic concept—a disease, disorder, injury, or health condition that can stand alone as a diagnosis. Stem codes are what most clinicians think of when they think of diagnostic codes: entities like 'Major depressive disorder, single episode' or 'Type 2 diabetes mellitus' or 'Chronic primary low back pain.'

A cluster code is a post-coordinated diagnostic expression: a stem code combined with one or more extension codes to create a more precise description. The cluster is the complete diagnostic statement, capturing not just what condition the patient has but relevant dimensions of that condition's presentation.

Consider again the clinical scenario of moderate chronic low back pain with significant functional limitation. In ICD-11, this would be expressed as a cluster combining MG30.01 (Chronic primary low back pain) as the stem code, XS25 (Moderate severity) as a severity extension, and XS9K (Significant functional limitation) as a functional impact extension.

The resulting cluster—MG30.01 & XS25 & XS9K—expresses the

complete clinical picture in structured, computable form. A researcher querying for chronic pain patients can identify this case. An analyst examining pain severity distributions can correctly classify it. A health system tracking functional outcomes can measure change over time. All of this was impossible with ICD-10, where the clinical detail existed only in narrative notes.

Post-coordination is governed by sanctioning rules embedded in the ICD-11 coding tool. These rules specify which extension codes can legitimately combine with which stem codes, preventing clinically nonsensical combinations while permitting the flexibility to capture clinical nuance. The rules are maintained as part of the Foundation, updated as clinical understanding evolves.

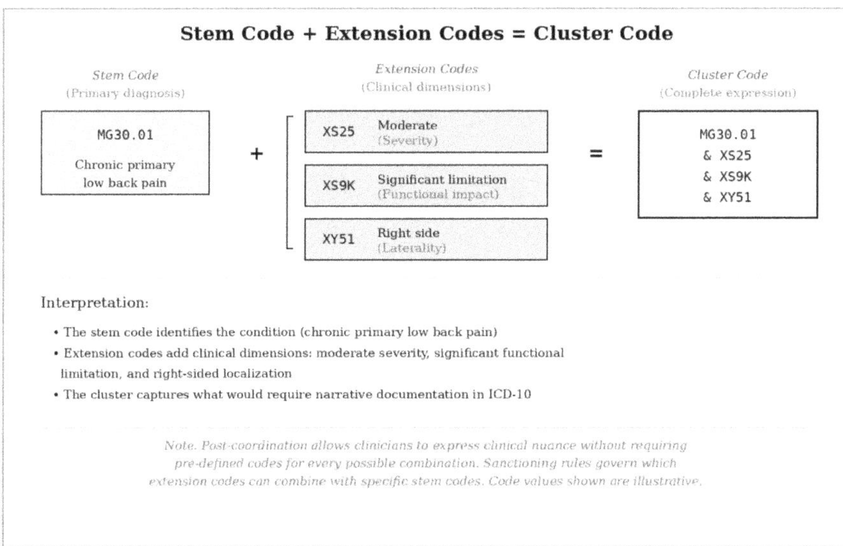

Figure 4.3. Stem and Cluster Code Relationship. The stem code identifies the primary diagnosis. Extension codes add clinical dimensions such as severity, functional impact, and laterality. The resulting cluster code captures the complete clinical picture in structured, computable form.

What This Architecture Enables

The architectural choices described in this chapter have practical consequences for how ICD-11 can serve clinical, research, and administrative purposes. Understanding these consequences helps clinicians appreciate why the system works as it does and what they can expect from it.

For clinical documentation, the architecture enables precision without proliferation. Clinicians can express detailed diagnostic descriptions without requiring the code set to anticipate every possible combination in advance. The documentation can be as specific as clinical knowledge warrants, with that specificity captured in structured data rather than lost in free text.

For research, the architecture enables cohort identification at multiple levels of granularity. Investigators can query broadly by stem code to capture all cases of a condition, or narrowly by post-coordinated clusters to identify cases with specific characteristics. The Foundation's semantic structure supports these queries in ways that a flat code list cannot.

For epidemiology and public health surveillance, the architecture enables tracking of conditions that previous systems could not adequately represent. When new conditions emerge or existing conditions are reconceptualized, the Foundation can be updated and new codes propagated without waiting for a full revision cycle. The response to COVID-19 demonstrated this capability, with emergency codes deployed rapidly within the ICD-11 framework.

For health information exchange, the architecture enables interoperability. Each entity's unique identifier persists across contexts, supporting data linkage and aggregation. The semantic structure supports mapping to other terminology systems, facilitating integration with electronic health records and health information exchanges that use different internal vocabularies.

What This Architecture Does Not Do

Clarity about the architecture also requires clarity about its limits. ICD-11's structural innovations do not extend to domains outside classification's proper scope, and understanding these boundaries prevents misplaced expectations.

The architecture does not mandate clinical decisions. A code describes what a clinician has diagnosed; it does not prescribe what treatment should follow. The availability of more precise diagnostic codes does not change the fundamental relationship between diagnosis and clinical judgment. Treatment decisions remain the province of clinicians applying their expertise to individual patients.

The architecture does not determine reimbursement. How payers use diagnostic codes, what payment rates attach to different diagnoses, and how coding affects revenue are matters of health policy and payer contracts, not classification design. ICD-11's greater expressiveness could support more nuanced payment models, but whether such models are adopted depends on decisions far outside the classification system itself.

The architecture does not guarantee data quality. Post-coordination enables precise documentation but does not ensure that clinicians will use it precisely. Extension codes can capture severity and functional impact but do not ensure that this information will be recorded. The system provides capacity; realizing that capacity depends on training, workflow integration, and institutional commitment to documentation quality.

The architecture does not eliminate the need for clinical expertise in coding. While ICD-11's digital tools provide more guidance than previous systems, the application of codes to clinical situations still requires understanding of both the clinical content and the classification logic. Automated coding assistance can support but not replace human judgment in complex cases.

Positioning for What Follows

The architecture described in this chapter provides the foundation for understanding the clinical domain chapters that follow. When Chapter 5 examines chronic pain classification, the discussion will reference how post-coordination enables documentation of pain severity, functional impact, and psychological dimensions. When Chapter 6 addresses autism and neurodevelopmental conditions, the analysis will show how specifiers for intellectual functioning and language capacity operate within the architectural framework described here.

Similarly, when later chapters address research implications and system preparation, they will build on the architectural concepts introduced in this chapter. The Foundation's structure determines what research queries are possible. The linearization model affects how countries can adapt the classification to local needs. Post-coordination influences what health information systems must support to fully utilize ICD-11's capabilities.

Readers need not memorize the technical details presented here. What matters is the conceptual understanding: ICD-11 is not merely a larger code list but a fundamentally different kind of classification system, built to represent clinical knowledge in ways that support both human comprehension and computational processing. This understanding provides context for everything that follows.

PART II

CLINICAL DOMAINS

5

CHRONIC PAIN

Chronic pain affects more people worldwide than any other health condition. The Global Burden of Disease studies consistently rank conditions characterized by chronic pain among the leading causes of years lived with disability. Low back pain alone accounts for more disability globally than any other condition. Yet for decades, the classification system that organizes how medicine names and categorizes disease had no coherent framework for representing chronic pain. Conditions were scattered across chapters, coded by anatomical location rather than clinical reality, and often forced into categories that implied either structural pathology or psychological disorder when neither fit the patient's experience.

ICD-11 changes this fundamentally. For the first time in the history of the International Classification of Diseases, chronic pain has a dedicated chapter built on contemporary pain science, developed through collaboration between the World Health Organization and the International Association for the Study of Pain. This chapter provides the diagnostic language that chronic pain has long lacked: language that recognizes chronic pain as a condition requiring attention in its own right, that distinguishes between pain arising from other diseases and pain that is itself the primary clinical problem, and that allows documentation of severity, mechanism, and functional impact.

This chapter examines what ICD-11 offers for chronic pain classification. It explains why reclassification was necessary, what the new categories contain, and how the system enables more precise clinical documentation. Throughout, the focus remains on classification rather than treatment. ICD-11 provides diagnostic language; it does not prescribe clinical pathways. Understanding this distinction is essential for appreciating what the new classification accomplishes and what it deliberately leaves to clinical judgment.

Why Chronic Pain Required Reclassification

The inadequacy of ICD-10 for chronic pain was structural, not merely a matter of missing codes. ICD-10 was designed when chronic pain was understood primarily as a symptom of underlying tissue pathology, and its architecture reflected that understanding. Pain codes appeared throughout the classification, attached to the organ systems where pain was perceived rather than organized according to the clinical characteristics of pain itself.

Consider how a clinician treating a patient with chronic low back pain navigated ICD-10. The available codes included M54.5 for low back pain in the musculoskeletal chapter, G89.29 for other chronic pain in the nervous system chapter, and F45.41 for pain disorder with psychological factors. None of these codes captured chronic low back pain as a coherent clinical entity. None allowed documentation of severity or functional impact. None distinguished between pain arising from identifiable structural pathology and pain that persisted despite the absence of proportionate findings.

This fragmentation had consequences beyond coding convenience. When chronic pain lacks coherent classification, epidemiological research becomes unreliable. Health policy decisions cannot be informed by prevalence data that does not exist. Resource allocation cannot address a burden that official statistics fail to capture. The conceptual limitation was equally significant: ICD-10's structure implied that pain was either the result of tissue damage or the result of psychological factors, leaving no room for pain maintained by changes in nervous system processing.

Research has increasingly demonstrated that structural findings often fail to explain chronic pain. A landmark study in the New England Journal of Medicine found that 64 percent of people with no back pain had disc bulges, protrusions, or herniations on MRI—structural changes that are common signs of normal aging rather than indicators of pain-causing pathology (Jensen et al., 1994). Subsequent research has consistently shown weak correlation between imaging abnormalities and pain symptoms, yet clinical practice continued to operate within a classification framework that implied structural causation.

Treede and colleagues articulated the problem that the IASP task force set out to address:

Chronic pain is a major source of suffering. It interferes with daily functioning and often is accompanied by distress. Yet, in the International Classification of Diseases, chronic pain diagnoses are not represented systematically. The lack of appropriate codes renders accurate epidemiological investigations difficult and impedes health policy decisions regarding chronic pain such as adequate financing of access to multimodal pain management. (Treede et al., 2019, p. 19)

Addressing these barriers required not merely adding codes but reconceptualizing how chronic pain should be represented within a classification system.

The IASP-WHO Collaboration

The chronic pain classification in ICD-11 emerged from a decade-long collaboration between the International Association for the Study of Pain and the World Health Organization. The IASP Task Force for the Classification of Chronic Pain, established in 2012, brought together pain specialists from across the globe to develop proposals that would then be integrated into the broader classification revision.

The task force faced a fundamental challenge: pain conditions are defined variously by perceived location, by etiology, by affected anatomical system, or by clinical pattern. Any classification scheme had to accommodate this heterogeneity while remaining clinically useful. The solution adopted prioritized etiology first, followed by underlying pathophysiological mechanisms, and finally body site. This hierarchical approach allowed the classification to accommodate different types of pain conditions while maintaining logical coherence.

Field testing at pain centers across multiple continents evaluated whether the categories were clinically useful, mutually exclusive, and exhaustive. Clinicians reported that the new categories captured clinical realities that previous classifications had missed.

Chronic Primary and Chronic Secondary Pain

The fundamental organizing principle of the ICD-11 chronic pain classification is the distinction between chronic primary pain and chronic secondary pain. This distinction reflects contemporary understanding that chronic pain can exist as a condition in its own right, not merely as a symptom of some other disease.

Chronic pain is defined throughout the classification as pain that persists or recurs for longer than three months. This duration threshold distinguishes chronic pain from acute pain, which serves a protective function by signaling tissue damage, and from subacute pain, which represents the transition period during normal healing.

Chronic primary pain is defined as chronic pain in one or more anatomical regions that is characterized by significant emotional distress or functional disability, and that cannot be better explained by another chronic pain condition. The key conceptual move here is recognizing that pain can be the primary clinical problem rather than a symptom pointing to something else. Conditions classified under chronic primary pain include chronic widespread pain such as fibromyalgia, chronic primary headache including migraine and tension-type headache, chronic primary visceral pain such as irritable bowel syndrome, and chronic primary musculoskeletal pain including chronic low back pain when not attributable to specific structural pathology.

Chronic secondary pain, by contrast, is chronic pain that arises as a symptom of an underlying condition. The underlying condition may be ongoing tissue pathology, nerve damage, or disease processes that generate pain through identifiable mechanisms. Chronic secondary pain categories include chronic cancer-related pain, chronic postsurgical and posttraumatic pain, chronic neuropathic pain, chronic secondary headache and orofacial pain, chronic secondary visceral pain, and chronic secondary musculoskeletal pain.

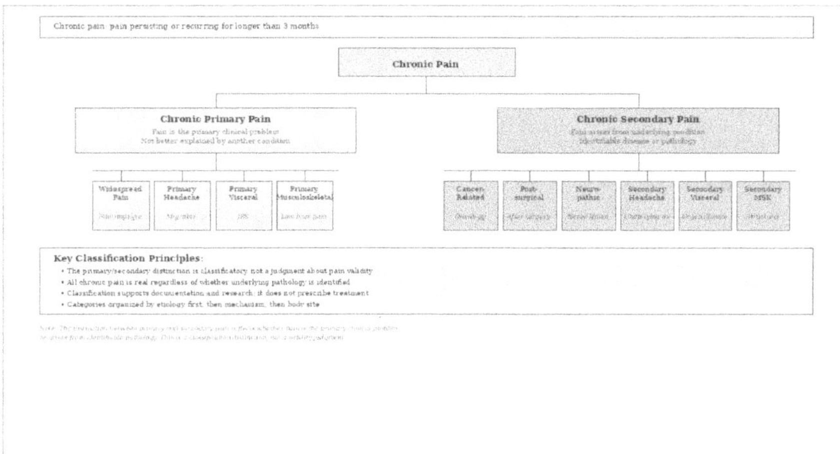

Figure 5.1. Chronic Pain Classification. ICD-11 distinguishes between chronic primary pain, where pain is the primary clinical problem, and chronic secondary pain, where pain arises from an identifiable underlying condition. All categories share the duration criterion of pain persisting or recurring for more than three months.

The distinction between primary and secondary pain is not a judgment about whether pain is real or legitimate. All chronic pain is real. The distinction is classificatory: it identifies whether the pain is best understood as arising from an identifiable underlying condition or whether the pain itself constitutes the primary clinical problem. This classification has implications for clinical documentation and research cohort identification, not for the validity of patient experience.

Table 5.1. Chronic Pain Codes: ICD-10 vs. ICD-11

CONDITION	ICD-10 APPROACH	ICD-11 APPROACH
Chronic low back pain	M54.5 (musculoskeletal) or G89.29 (chronic pain)	MG30.01 Chronic primary low back pain with severity/function codes
Fibromyalgia	M79.7 (soft tissue disorder)	MG30.0 Chronic widespread pain with extension codes
Chronic migraine	G43.7 (nervous system)	MG30.2 Chronic primary headache with mechanism descriptors
Cancer pain	Various codes by site; R52.1 chronic intractable	MG30.1 Chronic cancer-related pain with etiology link
Neuropathic pain	G89.29 or site-specific codes	MG30.5 Chronic neuropathic pain with mechanism specification
Post-surgical pain	No specific code; G89.28 other chronic postprocedural	MG30.2 Chronic postsurgical pain with temporal codes

Note: ICD-11 provides dedicated chronic pain categories with post-coordination capability, replacing fragmented ICD-10 codes that scattered pain across organ system chapters.

Mechanistic Descriptors and Nociplastic Pain

Beyond the categorical structure of chronic pain classification, ICD-11 incorporates mechanistic descriptors that allow clinicians to indicate the type of pain processing involved in a patient's presentation. These descriptors reflect advances in pain science that have moved beyond simple tissue-based models toward understanding of how the nervous system processes and modulates pain signals.

Three mechanistic descriptors are now recognized: nociceptive, neuropathic, and nociplastic. Each describes a different mechanism through which pain arises, and understanding these distinctions is important for appreciating what ICD-11's classification makes possible.

Nociceptive pain arises from actual or threatened damage to non-neural tissue and involves activation of nociceptors. This is the most familiar type of pain, corresponding to the common experience of pain from injury, inflammation, or mechanical stress on tissues. The pain is proportionate to the nature and extent of tissue involvement, and it resolves as the tissue heals.

Neuropathic pain is caused by a lesion or disease of the somatosensory nervous system. Unlike nociceptive pain, which involves normal function of the pain-sensing system in response to tissue damage, neuropathic pain involves abnormal function of the nervous system itself. Examples include pain following nerve injury, painful diabetic neuropathy, and postherpetic neuralgia.

Nociplastic pain is defined as pain arising from altered nociception despite no clear evidence of actual or threatened tissue damage causing activation of peripheral nociceptors, and despite no evidence for disease or lesion of the somatosensory system causing the pain. This term, adopted by the International Association for the Study of Pain in 2017, provides language for pain that cannot be fully explained by tissue pathology or nerve damage but that involves demonstrable changes in how the nervous system processes pain signals.

Recognition of nociplastic mechanisms reflects advances in neuroscience and pain processing, not a shift toward attributing pain to psychological causation. Neuroimaging research has demonstrated that chronic pain involves widespread changes in brain structure and function. In a striking example, researchers at Northwestern University tracked patients after an initial episode of back pain and predicted with 85 percent accuracy which patients would develop chronic pain based on brain scans alone—not by examining their backs (Baliki et al., 2012). When pain shifts from acute to chronic, it appears to move to brain regions involved in emotion, memory, and learning, suggesting that chronic pain is fundamentally a brain-learning phenomenon (Hashmi et al., 2013).

This neurobiological understanding does not reduce chronic pain to a psychological problem. It recognizes that pain processing involves the nervous system in complex ways that transcend simple tissue-damage models. Clinical research has shown that interventions targeting these neural processes can produce measurable changes in both brain function and pain experience, providing further evidence that the mechanisms underlying chronic pain are real, identifiable, and potentially modifiable.

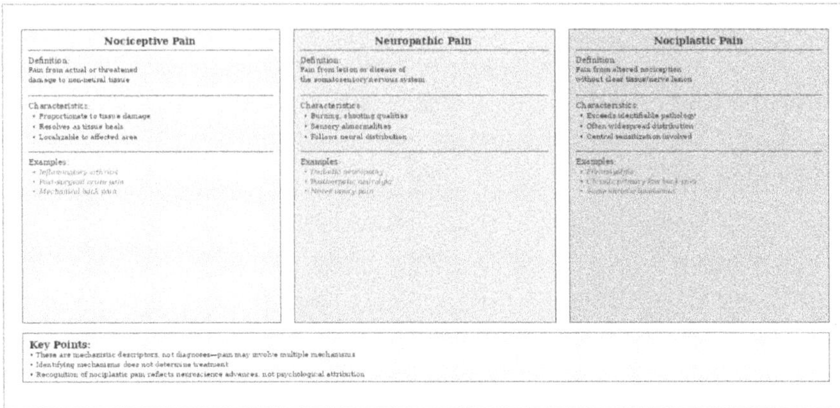

Figure 5.2. Pain Mechanism Subtypes. The three mechanistic descriptors—nociceptive, neuropathic, and nociplastic—describe different ways pain arises and is processed. These are not mutually exclusive; a patient's pain may involve multiple mechanisms.

Several clarifications about nociplastic pain are essential. First, nociplastic is a mechanistic descriptor, not a diagnosis. A patient does not receive a diagnosis of nociplastic pain; rather, their chronic pain condition may involve nociplastic mechanisms. Second, the mechanistic descriptors are not mutually exclusive. A patient may have pain with both nociceptive and nociplastic features, or neuropathic and nociplastic features. Pain conditions are often mixed in their mechanisms. Third, identifying nociplastic mechanisms does not determine treatment. The descriptor indicates what type of pain processing is likely involved; it does not prescribe what interventions are appropriate.

Post-coordination in Pain Diagnosis

The chronic pain classification gains additional power from ICD-11's post-coordination architecture described in Chapter 4. The ability to combine stem codes with extension codes allows pain diagnoses to express clinical detail that categorical codes alone cannot capture.

Consider the dimensions that matter clinically in chronic pain. Severity ranges from mild interference with function to complete disability. Temporal patterns may be constant, episodic, or fluctuating. Functional impact varies enormously across patients with the same diagnostic category. Under ICD-10, none of these dimensions could be captured systematically. A patient with severe, disabling chronic low back pain received the same code as a patient with mild, intermittent symptoms.

ICD-11's extension codes allow severity, temporal course, and pain-related functional impairment to accompany the diagnostic code. The result is a diagnostic expression that captures what the clinician observes rather than forcing clinical reality into predetermined categories. This expressiveness has particular value for chronic pain because of the heterogeneity within diagnostic categories—two patients with fibromyalgia may present very differently in severity, predominant symptoms, and functional impact.

These findings underscore why classification that reflects pain mechanisms matters: diagnostic language shapes which forms of care are considered legitimate and appropriate. When severity and functional impact can be coded systematically, investigators can stratify cohorts by these dimensions rather than treating heterogeneous populations as uniform. Treatment response can be analyzed in relation to documented baseline characteristics. Longitudinal changes can be tracked through structured data rather than inferred from clinical notes.

What This Classification Does and Does Not Do

Clarity about the scope and limits of the chronic pain classification is essential for appropriate use. The classification is a tool for systematic representation of clinical phenomena. It is not a guide to clinical decision-making, and it should not be treated as one.

The classification provides diagnostic categories that represent chronic pain as a legitimate clinical domain. For the first time, clinicians have codes that acknowledge chronic pain as a condition requiring attention rather than merely a symptom to be traced to something else. It allows documentation of severity, temporal pattern, and functional impact. It incorporates mechanistic descriptors that reflect contemporary pain science.

What the classification does not do is equally important. It does not determine etiology conclusively—a diagnosis of chronic primary low back pain indicates that the pain is not better explained by an identifiable secondary cause, not what is causing the pain. It does not dictate treatment; the classification describes conditions but does not prescribe interventions. It does not invalidate structural or pathological findings; the existence of chronic primary pain categories does not mean clinicians should stop looking for treatable causes.

Critically, the classification does not imply that pain is psychological when structural causes are not identified. The chronic primary pain categories represent pain as a clinical phenomenon, not as evidence of psychological disorder. These boundaries matter because classification systems can be misused. The IASP task force was explicit that the classification was designed to improve recognition and documentation of chronic pain, not to provide ammunition for denying its reality.

Implications and the Path Forward

The availability of coherent chronic pain classification in ICD-11 has implications extending beyond individual clinical documentation. For research, cohort identification becomes more reliable when chronic pain conditions have consistent diagnostic representation. For epidemiological surveillance, prevalence estimates become possible when the classification system provides adequate codes. For health system planning, resource allocation for chronic pain services depends on understanding how many people are affected and what types of chronic pain predominate.

Emerging research demonstrates why accurate classification matters for treatment development. A randomized controlled trial published in JAMA Psychiatry found that 66 percent of patients with chronic back pain were nearly or fully pain-free after a psychological intervention that taught patients to reinterpret pain signals as nonthreatening, compared to only 10 percent in the control group—with results maintained at one-year follow-up (Ashar et al., 2022). Such findings underscore that when classification accurately reflects pain mechanisms, it opens pathways to interventions that might otherwise seem implausible within a purely structural framework.

The recognition of chronic pain as a legitimate diagnostic domain also has implications for clinical legitimacy. Patients with chronic pain have often struggled for recognition within health systems that treated their conditions as either manifestations of undiscovered pathology or as psychological problems. A classification that represents chronic pain as a clinical domain in its own right supports the legitimacy of chronic pain populations without prejudging what is causing any individual's pain.

The chapters that follow examine other clinical domains where ICD-11 offers substantial improvements. Chapter 6 addresses autism and neurodevelopmental conditions, where similar issues of heterogeneity and inadequate classification have created parallel challenges. Chapter 7 examines post-viral syndromes. Chapter 8 reviews updates in mental and behavioral health classification.

For clinicians who have worked for years without adequate diagnostic language, this change matters. ICD-11 does not solve chronic pain, but it finally names it accurately. That alone reshapes what research can ask, what systems can see, and what patients can be recognized.

6

AUTISM AND NEURODEVELOPMENT

Few areas of clinical classification have generated as much discussion as the classification of autism and related neurodevelopmental conditions. The stakes are substantial: classification shapes who receives diagnoses, how services are organized, what research cohorts look like, and how individuals understand their own developmental histories. For decades, clinicians and researchers worked within classification frameworks that subdivided the autism spectrum into discrete categories, imposed childhood-specific assumptions on conditions that persist across the lifespan, and struggled to accommodate the heterogeneity that characterizes neurodevelopmental presentations.

ICD-11 approaches neurodevelopmental conditions differently. Rather than maintaining artificial boundaries between subtypes that clinical experience and research evidence could not reliably distinguish, the new classification consolidates autism into a single spectrum diagnosis with dimensional specifiers. Rather than assuming that neurodevelopmental conditions are primarily childhood phenomena, it adopts a lifespan orientation that acknowledges adult identification and changing functional demands across development. Rather than forcing clinicians to choose single diagnoses when multiple neurodevelopmental conditions co-occur, it permits documentation of the complex profiles that many individuals present.

This chapter examines how ICD-11 classifies autism and other neurodevelopmental conditions. It explains why reclassification was necessary, what the new framework contains, how dimensional description works within it, and what the classification does and does not accomplish. Throughout, the focus remains on classification logic rather than on treatment approaches or identity frameworks.

Why Neurodevelopmental Conditions Required Reclassification

The classification of autism and related conditions in ICD-10 reflected the scientific understanding of its era. The Pervasive Developmental Disorders category included childhood autism, atypical autism, Rett syndrome, other childhood disintegrative disorder, Asperger syndrome, and several residual categories. This structure implied that these were distinct conditions with different etiologies, courses, and clinical implications.

Clinical experience and accumulating research evidence challenged this categorical architecture. The boundaries between childhood autism and Asperger syndrome proved impossible to draw reliably. Clinicians in different settings, applying ostensibly the same criteria, reached different conclusions about which category applied to a given individual. Research attempting to validate the distinction through genetic, neuroimaging, or outcome studies failed to identify consistent biological or prognostic markers that separated the putative subtypes.

The consequences of this diagnostic instability were substantial. Epidemiological estimates varied wildly depending on whether studies used narrow or broad definitions. Service eligibility often depended on which specific diagnosis an individual received, creating arbitrary disparities in access to support. Research cohorts assembled under one diagnostic label might differ fundamentally from cohorts assembled under another, compromising comparability of findings across studies.

Beyond the subtype problem, ICD-10's framing of neurodevelopmental conditions as primarily childhood disorders created additional limitations. The classification provided no clear pathway for identifying autism in adults who had not been diagnosed in childhood. As awareness increased and understanding of how autism presents differently across age, gender, and context expanded, growing numbers of adults sought evaluation for conditions that had shaped their lives but had never been formally recognized.

Reed and colleagues, describing the principles guiding the ICD-11 revision, articulated the broader goals that shaped the neurodevelopmental classification:

The development of the ICD-11 CDDG over the past decade, based on the principles of clinical utility and global applicability, has been the most broadly international, multilingual, multidisciplinary and participative revision process ever implemented for a classification of mental disorders. Innovations in the ICD-11 include the provision of consistent and systematically characterized information, the adoption of a lifespan approach, and culture-related guidance for each disorder. (Reed et al., 2019, p. 3)

ICD-11's Neurodevelopmental Framework

ICD-11 consolidates neurodevelopmental conditions into a coherent diagnostic grouping positioned at the beginning of the chapter on Mental, Behavioural and Neurodevelopmental Disorders. This placement reflects the developmental perspective that organizes the entire chapter, proceeding from conditions with origins in early development through conditions more characteristic of later life.

The neurodevelopmental disorders grouping includes disorders of intellectual development, developmental speech or language disorders, autism spectrum disorder, developmental learning disorder, developmental motor coordination disorder, attention deficit hyperactivity disorder, stereotyped movement disorder, and a category for other specified and unspecified neurodevelopmental disorders. These conditions share several conceptual features: onset during the developmental period, patterns that affect multiple domains of functioning, and courses that extend across the lifespan even as manifestations change.

The reorganization removes conditions that had been grouped with neurodevelopmental disorders in ICD-10 but that subsequent evidence suggested belonged elsewhere. Rett syndrome, now understood as a specific genetic condition with a known etiology, is classified with diseases of the nervous system rather than with behaviorally defined neurodevelopmental conditions.

Autism Spectrum Disorder as a Dimensional Diagnosis

The most significant change in the autism classification is the consolidation of previously separate diagnoses into a single category: Autism Spectrum Disorder. This category encompasses what ICD-10 classified as childhood autism, atypical autism, Asperger syndrome, and other pervasive developmental disorders. The consolidation reflects recognition that these presentations represent variation along a spectrum rather than categorically distinct conditions.

The ICD-11 description of Autism Spectrum Disorder identifies persistent deficits in initiating and sustaining reciprocal social interaction and social communication, together with restricted, repetitive, and inflexible patterns of behavior, interests, or activities. These core features must be present from early in the developmental period, though they may not become fully manifest until social demands exceed the individual's capacity to manage them.

Rather than subdividing autism into categorical subtypes, ICD-11 uses dimensional specifiers to characterize individual presentations. Two specifiers are particularly important: intellectual development and functional language. For intellectual development, clinicians indicate whether the individual has a co-occurring disorder of intellectual development and, if so, at what level of severity. For functional language, clinicians indicate whether functional language is present and, if so, to what degree.

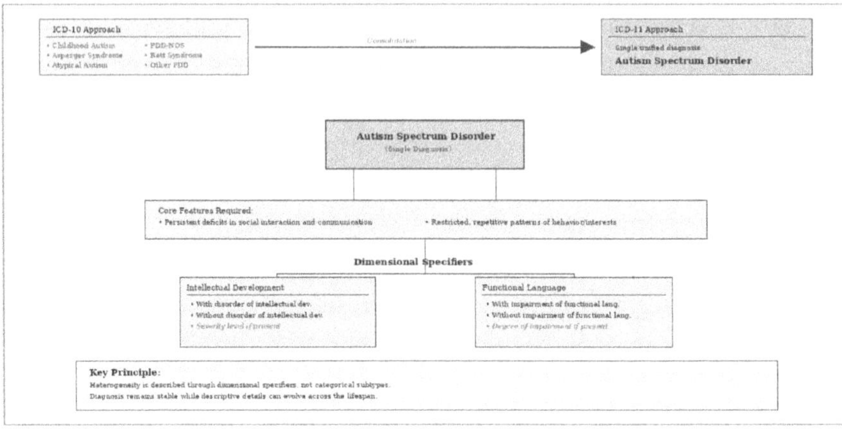

Figure 6.1. Autism Dimensional Model. ICD-11 consolidates multiple ICD-10 subtypes into a single Autism Spectrum Disorder diagnosis. Heterogeneity is captured through dimensional specifiers rather than categorical distinctions.

This dimensional approach accommodates heterogeneity without fragmenting the spectrum into categories that lack empirical support. Two individuals with Autism Spectrum Disorder may present very differently: one with intact intellectual development and fluent functional language, another with significant intellectual disability and minimal spoken language. The dimensional specifiers capture this variation while maintaining the conceptual unity of the spectrum. This approach is supported by extensive research demonstrating shared etiological factors across presentations that were previously classified separately (Lai et al., 2014; Lord et al., 2018).

Table 6.1. Autism Classification: ICD-10 vs. ICD-11

FEATURE	ICD-10	ICD-11
Diagnostic structure	Categorical subtypes (Childhood Autism, Asperger, Atypical, etc.)	Unified spectrum with dimensional specifiers
Developmental frame	Childhood-focused terminology and criteria	Lifespan orientation; adult identification recognized
Co-occurrence	Discouraged ADHD co-diagnosis; forced primary choice	Permits multiple co-occurring diagnoses
Diagnostic stability	Subtype reclassification common across life stages	Diagnosis stable; specifiers track changes
Functional description	Limited to category selection	Specifiers for intellectual dev. and language

Note: The ICD-11 approach addresses empirical challenges with subtype distinctions while providing structured description of individual variation through dimensional specifiers.

Diagnostic Stability Over Time

One underappreciated consequence of the ICD-11 approach is improved diagnostic stability over time. Under ICD-10, individuals were often reclassified as they aged, moved between systems, or encountered different evaluators—not because their underlying neurodevelopmental profile had changed, but because the available categories forced different interpretive choices at different stages of life.

The unified spectrum model with dimensional specifiers allows the diagnosis itself to remain stable while the descriptive details evolve. An individual diagnosed with Autism Spectrum Disorder in childhood retains that diagnosis into adulthood; what may change are the specifiers describing intellectual development, functional language, or other dimensional features. This supports continuity of care, reduces administrative disruption, and preserves the integrity of longitudinal clinical records.

For electronic health records and research datasets, this stability matters considerably. When diagnoses shift between categorical subtypes across evaluations, linking records becomes unreliable and longitudinal tracking becomes difficult. A classification system that maintains diagnostic continuity while allowing descriptive evolution creates cleaner data and more coherent clinical histories.

Lifespan Orientation and Late Identification

ICD-11 explicitly acknowledges that autism and other neurodevelopmental conditions extend across the entire lifespan. While onset occurs during the developmental period, the classification recognizes that features may not become fully manifest until later, when social demands exceed the individual's capacities. This recognition has profound implications for how clinicians approach assessment in adolescents and adults.

The ICD-11 Clinical Descriptions and Diagnostic Guidelines note that some individuals with Autism Spectrum Disorder function adequately in many contexts through exceptional effort, such that their differences may not be apparent to others or may only emerge under specific circumstances. Social demands change across development: the relatively structured environment of childhood gives way to the more complex social navigation required in adolescence and adulthood.

This lifespan orientation matters for several reasons. It legitimizes adult identification rather than treating late diagnosis as inherently suspect. It provides a framework for understanding why some individuals reach adulthood without a diagnosis despite having had autism throughout their lives. It acknowledges that autism is not a condition one outgrows but rather a developmental pattern whose expression changes as the individual and their context change.

The ICD-11 framework also supports the growing recognition of adult autism services as a legitimate and necessary component of healthcare systems, rather than an extension of pediatric models that many adults never accessed.

Co-occurrence and Diagnostic Expressiveness

Neurodevelopmental conditions frequently co-occur—not as exceptions but as the modal presentation in many clinical settings. An individual may meet criteria for both Autism Spectrum Disorder and Attention Deficit Hyperactivity Disorder. Autism Spectrum Disorder commonly co-occurs with disorders of intellectual development. Multiple neurodevelopmental conditions may be present alongside anxiety disorders, mood disorders, or other mental health conditions.

ICD-10 created barriers to documenting this co-occurrence. The classification of autism and ADHD, for example, was complicated by guidance that discouraged assigning both diagnoses to the same individual. Clinicians faced pressure to choose a primary diagnosis even when both conditions were clearly present and clinically significant. This forced choice distorted clinical documentation and compromised the accuracy of research cohorts.

ICD-11 permits co-occurring diagnoses when multiple conditions are present. An individual can receive diagnoses of Autism Spectrum Disorder and Attention Deficit Hyperactivity Disorder without artificial hierarchy or exclusion. The dimensional specifiers for autism further enable documentation of co-occurring intellectual disability within the autism diagnosis itself.

From a systems perspective, recognizing co-occurrence as typical rather than exceptional has implications for workforce planning and service design. Models built around single-diagnosis pathways may fail to serve the actual patient population effectively. Multidisciplinary care, coordinated services, and training that addresses complex presentations become necessities rather than luxuries when the classification system accurately reflects clinical reality.

Clinical Consequences of Dimensional Classification

Dimensional classification changes how autism is documented without changing the threshold for diagnosis. Clinicians no longer need to decide whether an individual fits a subtype; instead, they describe the individual's functional profile within a shared diagnostic framework. This reduces artificial diagnostic variation across settings and providers, improves communication between disciplines, and allows documentation to track meaningful change over time without redefining the underlying condition.

From a systems perspective, this shift matters because services, accommodations, and research eligibility often hinge on diagnostic labels. A classification system that produces inconsistent labels for similar presentations undermines equity and continuity. ICD-11's dimensional approach addresses this by separating the question of whether autism is present from the question of how it presents in this individual at this time.

For clinicians who work in workflows—schools, disability services, insurance authorization—the practical consequence is reduced diagnostic churn. When the diagnostic label remains stable and only descriptive specifiers change, administrative processes that depend on diagnosis are less likely to be disrupted by re-evaluation. This represents a genuine improvement in clinical utility.

What This Classification Does and Does Not Do

Clarity about the scope and limits of the neurodevelopmental classification is essential for appropriate use. The classification provides diagnostic categories based on current scientific understanding and clinical consensus. It consolidates autism into a spectrum diagnosis with dimensional specifiers. It adopts a lifespan orientation that recognizes adult identification. It permits documentation of co-occurring conditions.

What the classification does not do is equally important to understand. It does not define identity. Whether an individual considers their autism a disorder, a disability, a difference, or a central aspect of who they are is not determined by the classification system. The classification provides diagnostic language; it does not prescribe how individuals should understand or relate to their diagnoses.

The classification does not dictate support models or intervention approaches. The longstanding debates about behavioral interventions, educational approaches, support philosophies, and therapeutic orientations are not resolved by how conditions are classified. Classification is prior to and separate from questions about what should be done once a condition is identified.

The classification does not erase disability. The dimensional approach to autism does not imply that autism is merely a difference without functional implications. The diagnostic criteria explicitly require that features cause impairment in important areas of functioning. Recognizing autism as a spectrum does not minimize the substantial support needs of many autistic individuals.

Implications for Research and Health Systems

The changes in neurodevelopmental classification have implications that extend beyond individual clinical encounters. For research, the consolidation of autism subtypes into a single spectrum diagnosis changes how cohorts are defined. Studies can no longer compare Asperger syndrome to childhood autism as distinct populations; the distinction no longer exists. Instead, research can use dimensional specifiers to define cohorts based on intellectual development, functional language, or other characteristics.

Health system planning benefits from classification that captures clinical complexity. When co-occurring conditions can be documented systematically, planners can better understand what service configurations are needed. When dimensional specifiers indicate levels of intellectual development and functional language, resource allocation can reflect actual support needs rather than categorical assumptions.

International comparability improves when countries use the same classification system with the same diagnostic concepts. As ICD-11 achieves global adoption, research and surveillance data from different countries become more directly comparable, reducing one source of cross-national incomparability.

Positioning for What Follows

The classification of autism and neurodevelopmental conditions in ICD-11 represents a significant reconceptualization. The shift from categorical subtypes to a dimensional spectrum, the adoption of a lifespan orientation, and the permission to document co-occurring conditions all reflect accumulated evidence about how these conditions actually present across diverse populations and developmental stages.

These changes in classification do not resolve the many debates that surround autism and neurodevelopmental conditions. Questions about etiology, intervention, educational approach, and service organization remain active areas of discussion. The classification provides a framework for documenting and communicating about these conditions; it does not adjudicate the contested questions that concern researchers, clinicians, individuals, and families.

The chapters that follow examine other areas where ICD-11 offers significant advances. Chapter 7 addresses post-viral syndromes and related conditions, including the Long COVID presentations that have created urgent clinical and classificatory challenges. Chapter 8 reviews updates in mental and behavioral health classification.

For clinicians who work with individuals across the neurodevelopmental spectrum, the message of this chapter parallels that of Chapter 5: classification is catching up with clinical reality. The diagnostic language now available better reflects the heterogeneity, the lifespan course, and the co-occurrence patterns that characterize neurodevelopmental presentations. Using this language well requires understanding not only what the classification contains but also what it is and is not designed to accomplish.

7

POST-VIRAL SYNDROMES

Post-viral syndromes did not emerge with COVID-19. What emerged was the inability of existing classification systems to represent them. For decades, clinicians recognized that some patients failed to recover fully from acute infections, experiencing persistent fatigue, cognitive dysfunction, autonomic instability, and pain that existing diagnostic frameworks could not coherently express. The conditions were real. The classification was absent.

Long COVID did not create a new clinical phenomenon. It validated the existence of post-viral syndromes at a scale large enough to force classification reform. When millions of patients worldwide experienced persistent symptoms following SARS-CoV-2 infection, health systems could no longer treat post-infectious illness as an afterthought or an anomaly. The pandemic exposed a structural gap in how medicine names and tracks conditions defined by functional impairment rather than discrete pathology.

ICD-11 represents the first classification framework capable of expressing post-viral illness as a coherent, multi-system condition without presuming mechanism or assigning psychogenic causation.

This chapter examines how that framework operates, why it matters, and what it does and does not accomplish.

Classification Is Not Etiology

Before examining the specific codes and structures, one distinction requires emphasis. ICD-11 does not assert a single cause for post-viral syndromes. It does not privilege immune, autonomic, metabolic, neurological, or psychological explanations. Its contribution is more fundamental: it provides a framework for naming and tracking a clinical pattern that exists regardless of mechanism.

Classification precedes explanation. Without coherent classification, etiological research cannot progress—cohorts cannot be assembled, prevalence cannot be estimated, and interventions cannot be evaluated against appropriate comparators. The ICD-11 framework for post-viral syndromes establishes the descriptive foundation that mechanistic research requires. It does not claim to have solved the mechanistic questions that remain under active investigation.

Why Post-Viral Syndromes Challenged Prior Classification

Post-viral syndromes presented classification challenges long before the term entered common usage. Patients who failed to recover from acute infections often found their persistent symptoms scattered across multiple diagnostic categories or, worse, dismissed as unexplained. The classification problem was structural, not merely a matter of missing codes.

ICD-10 organized conditions primarily by etiology or affected organ system. Acute infections appeared under infectious diseases. Their consequences might appear under neurological conditions, cardiovascular disorders, or mental and behavioral categories, depending on which symptoms predominated. The connection between the triggering infection and the subsequent syndrome was not readily expressible within the classification structure itself.

This fragmentation had consequences. Epidemiological surveillance could not easily track post-infectious conditions because they lacked unified representation. Research cohorts assembled under one code might differ substantially from those assembled under another, despite describing clinically similar patients. Clinicians documenting the same syndrome might select different codes depending on their specialty, their institution's coding practices, or which symptom happened to prompt the clinical encounter.

The Cost of Diagnostic Invisibility

When conditions cannot be named coherently, the harm is cumulative. Patients cycle through specialties without unifying explanation. Research cohorts fragment. Surveillance undercounts prevalence. Interventions are evaluated against inappropriate comparators. Over time, the absence of classification becomes mistaken for absence of disease.

The problem was compounded by conditions whose primary manifestation was functional impairment rather than discrete pathology. A patient experiencing persistent fatigue, cognitive difficulties, and exercise intolerance following viral infection did not fit neatly into organ-based categories. The symptoms were real and disabling, but the classification system lacked adequate vocabulary for conditions defined by functional limitation rather than identifiable lesions. The diagnostic invisibility was not a judgment about the patients; it was a limitation of the classification system.

Historical Context: Post-Infectious Illness Before COVID-19

The classification challenges exposed by Long COVID were not novel. Several well-recognized conditions had already demonstrated that some infections leave lasting functional impairment that resists categorization under conventional diagnostic frameworks.

Myalgic encephalomyelitis/chronic fatigue syndrome represents perhaps the most extensively studied post-infectious condition predating COVID-19. While not all cases follow identifiable infections, a substantial proportion of patients report onset following acute viral illness. The condition is characterized by persistent fatigue not attributable to ongoing exertion, post-exertional malaise, unrefreshing sleep, and cognitive difficulties. Despite decades of research, its pathophysiology remains incompletely understood, and its classification has been contested across multiple revisions of diagnostic systems.

Post-polio syndrome provided an earlier example of delayed

consequences following acute infection. Patients who had recovered from acute poliomyelitis sometimes experienced new weakness, fatigue, and pain decades after their initial illness. Epstein-Barr virus and other herpesviruses have been associated with prolonged fatigue states following acute infection. These cases accumulated in clinical practice without finding adequate representation in classification systems designed around acute illness models.

Long COVID as a Classification Stress Test

The COVID-19 pandemic created conditions that made the classification gap impossible to ignore. The scale of infection, the visibility of persistent symptoms, and the urgency of public health response combined to demand classificatory attention that earlier post-infectious syndromes had not received.

Within months of the pandemic's onset, clinicians began reporting patients whose symptoms persisted well beyond the acute infection period. These patients did not fit the expected recovery trajectory. Some had been hospitalized with severe acute illness; others had experienced mild initial infections. The common feature was persistent, often fluctuating symptoms that impaired function across multiple domains.

The World Health Organization recognized the need for formal classification relatively early in the pandemic's course. A clinical case definition was developed through Delphi consensus, establishing criteria that could guide both clinical recognition and research cohort identification. Soriano and colleagues published this consensus definition:

Post COVID-19 condition occurs in individuals with a history of probable or confirmed SARS-CoV-2 infection, usually 3 months from the onset of COVID-19, with symptoms that last for at least 2 months and cannot be explained by an alternative diagnosis. Common symptoms include fatigue, shortness of breath, cognitive dysfunction but also others which generally have an impact on everyday functioning. (Soriano et al., 2022, p. 1173)

This definition accomplished several classificatory tasks simultaneously. It established temporal criteria, acknowledged symptom heterogeneity, specified functional impact as defining, and explicitly required exclusion of alternative diagnoses. The linguistic precision reflects appropriate epistemic humility in the face of a condition whose mechanisms continue to be studied.

ICD-11 Framework for Post-Viral Syndromes

ICD-11 provides specific codes for post COVID-19 condition and a broader framework for representing post-viral syndromes generally. The classification approach reflects lessons learned from earlier attempts to accommodate conditions defined by functional impairment rather than discrete pathology.

The code RA02 designates Post COVID-19 condition within the supplementary chapter for codes for special purposes. This placement acknowledges the condition's relationship to a specific pathogen while providing a stable identifier for documentation, surveillance, and research. The code can be used alongside other codes that capture specific manifestations, allowing comprehensive documentation of heterogeneous presentations.

The introduction of a linking code represents a conceptual departure from symptom-based coding. Rather than fragmenting post-viral illness into disconnected manifestations, ICD-11 preserves the relationship between the triggering infection and downstream effects while allowing full expression of heterogeneity. This structure resolves a longstanding tension between specificity and coherence that ICD-10 could not address.

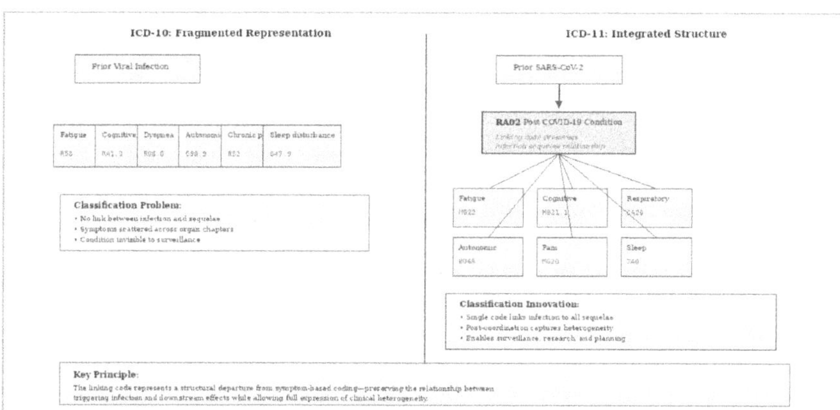

Figure 7.1. Post-Viral Syndrome Classification. ICD-10 fragmented post-viral symptoms across organ-based chapters with no linking structure. ICD-11's RA02 code preserves the infection-sequelae relationship while enabling post-coordination for heterogeneous manifestations.

Table 7.1. Post-Viral Syndrome Classification: ICD-10 vs. ICD-11

CHALLENGE	ICD-10 LIMITATION	ICD-11 SOLUTION
Heterogeneous symptoms	Scattered across organ chapters; no unified code	RA02 links all manifestations to triggering infection
Uncertain mechanism	Classification implied structural etiology	Classification agnostic to mechanism; descriptive
Temporal unpredictability	No accommodation for fluctuating course	Current status documentation; no prognosis required
Surveillance invisibility	Prevalence uncountable without unified code	Single code enables population monitoring
Multi-system involvement	Required separate codes per organ system	Post-coordination captures full presentation

Note. *The ICD-11 approach addresses classification failures that had rendered post-viral syndromes invisible to surveillance, fragmented in research, and inconsistent in clinical documentation.*

Functional Impact and Longitudinal Uncertainty

Post-viral syndromes challenge classification systems not only through their symptom heterogeneity but through their temporal unpredictability. Symptoms may fluctuate, relapse, partially resolve, or evolve over time. A classification designed for conditions with predictable trajectories must accommodate this uncertainty without abandoning its descriptive function.

The emphasis on functional impact addresses this challenge. Regardless of which symptoms predominate at any given time, the classification captures whether everyday functioning is impaired. This functional focus aligns with broader trends in health classification that recognize disability as central to what makes health conditions clinically significant.

The longitudinal uncertainty inherent in post-viral syndromes requires particular clinical attention. Some patients recover fully, though on timescales longer than acute illness models anticipate. Others experience persistent impairment. Still others follow relapsing courses that defy simple categorization. The classification accommodates this uncertainty by focusing on current functional status rather than requiring prognostic claims.

A diagnosis of post COVID-19 condition describes the patient's current state without implying permanence or recovery. The classification can be applied, maintained, or discontinued as the patient's status evolves. This flexibility acknowledges that clinicians must document what they observe while remaining uncertain about what comes next.

What This Classification Does and Does Not Do

Clarity about the scope of classification is essential when addressing conditions as contested and consequential as post-viral syndromes. The ICD-11 framework provides specific functions while explicitly declining to address questions beyond its classificatory mandate.

The classification does provide a recognized diagnostic category based on current scientific consensus. This recognition has practical consequences: it enables systematic documentation, supports epidemiological surveillance, facilitates research cohort identification, and provides a framework for health system planning. The existence of a code does not prove anything about mechanism or etiology, but it does establish that the condition exists as a clinically recognized entity.

The classification does not define mechanism. How SARS-CoV-2 or other viruses produce persistent symptoms remains under active investigation. Multiple hypotheses exist, including viral persistence, autoimmune phenomena, microvascular dysfunction, and nervous system involvement. The classification remains agnostic among these possibilities because classification serves documentation, not causal explanation.

The classification does not prescribe treatment. What interventions help patients with post-viral syndromes remains an active area of clinical research. The existence of a diagnostic code does not imply that specific treatments are indicated, effective, or reimbursable.

The classification does not imply psychogenic origin. The placement of functional impact at the center of the definition reflects what matters clinically, not an assertion about mechanism. Patients with post-viral syndromes report real symptoms with measurable functional consequences. The classification documents these observations without prejudging their etiology.

Research and Health System Implications

The classificatory changes described in this chapter have implications for research design, epidemiological surveillance, and health system planning. These implications extend beyond the immediate context of Long COVID to inform how health systems approach post-infectious conditions generally.

For research, the existence of standardized diagnostic criteria enables more consistent cohort identification. Studies using the WHO case definition will assemble more comparable patient groups than studies using idiosyncratic inclusion criteria. This comparability supports evidence synthesis, meta-analysis, and the accumulation of knowledge across research settings and populations.

For epidemiological surveillance, standardized classification enables population-level monitoring. Health systems can track incidence, prevalence, and temporal trends using consistent case definitions. International comparability improves when countries use the same classification system.

For health system planning, the classification provides vocabulary for describing service needs. How many patients require rehabilitation services, specialty consultation, or disability accommodation becomes answerable when consistent diagnostic categories are applied. The experience with Long COVID may inform how health systems respond to future post-infectious conditions—demonstrating that classification systems can adapt more rapidly than their historical revision cycles suggested.

Positioning for What Follows

The post-viral syndromes examined in this chapter represent a particular kind of classification challenge: conditions recognized clinically before their mechanisms are fully understood, characterized by functional impairment rather than discrete pathology, and following temporal patterns that resist simple categorization. ICD-11's framework for these conditions demonstrates classification proceeding under uncertainty, providing useful vocabulary while acknowledging the limits of current knowledge.

This approach parallels the classification strategies examined in earlier chapters. Chronic pain required recognition as a condition in its own right, not merely a symptom of something else. Autism spectrum disorder required dimensional specification rather than categorical fragmentation. Post-viral syndromes require accommodation of heterogeneity and longitudinal uncertainty without abandoning classificatory precision.

Once a condition is classifiable, it cannot be unseen. ICD-11 does not resolve the causes of post-viral syndromes, but it ensures they can be counted, studied, and addressed without distortion. That shift—from fragmentation to coherence—marks a permanent change in how medicine recognizes post-infectious illness.

Chapter 8 continues the examination of ICD-11's clinical domain changes by addressing mental and behavioral health. The classification changes in that domain reflect both scientific advances and evolving understanding of how psychological and behavioral conditions should be represented.

8

MENTAL AND BEHAVIORAL HEALTH

Mental and behavioral health has always presented distinctive classification challenges. The conditions grouped under this heading are defined primarily by patterns of experience and behavior rather than laboratory findings or imaging results. Their boundaries with normal variation are often contested. Their overlap with one another is substantial. Their causes remain, in most cases, incompletely understood. These features do not make mental and behavioral conditions less real or less important than other health conditions. They do make classification particularly consequential, because the categories themselves shape clinical thinking, research design, and service organization.

ICD-11 does not attempt to resolve debates about the nature of mental illness. It addresses a more fundamental problem: that prior classification systems created artificial boundaries, unstable diagnoses, and documentation practices that failed to reflect how mental and behavioral conditions actually present in clinical settings. The changes described in this chapter respond to these structural limitations while remaining agnostic about deeper theoretical questions that classification cannot answer.

This chapter examines the structural reorganization of mental and behavioral health classification in ICD-11. The goal is to explain what changed, why those changes were made, and what the changes enable for clinical documentation and research. This is an explanation of taxonomy, not an argument about theory.

Why Mental and Behavioral Health Required Reclassification

ICD-10's chapter on mental and behavioural disorders served clinical and research purposes for three decades. During that time, accumulated experience revealed structural limitations that affected diagnostic reliability, research comparability, and clinical utility across diverse settings.

The categorical structure of ICD-10 created artificial boundaries between conditions that shared substantial features. Anxiety and depression, for example, were classified as separate categories despite their frequent co-occurrence and overlapping symptom profiles. Clinicians regularly encountered patients who met criteria for multiple disorders simultaneously, raising questions about whether these represented genuinely distinct conditions or artifacts of categorical classification.

Diagnostic instability across settings and over time created problems for epidemiology and research. The same patient might receive different diagnoses depending on which symptoms were most prominent at a given assessment, which clinician conducted the evaluation, or which diagnostic tradition predominated in a particular setting. This instability compromised the comparability of research cohorts and complicated longitudinal tracking.

Beyond Categorical Absolutes

ICD-10 encouraged an implicit binary: either a patient had a disorder or did not; either symptoms fit a category or they did not. Clinical reality has never conformed to this logic. Two patients meeting criteria for the same diagnosis may differ dramatically in severity, functional impact, and treatment needs.

ICD-11's dimensional elements do not blur the distinction between disorder and normal variation. They allow clinicians to describe how much, in what way, and with what impact a condition is present once diagnostic threshold is met. The threshold remains meaningful. What changes is the capacity to describe variation above that threshold rather than treating all cases as equivalent.

Consider two patients who meet criteria for Major Depressive Disorder. One presents with mild symptoms and minimal functional impairment; the other presents with severe symptoms, impaired occupational functioning, and suicidality. Under ICD-10, both receive the same diagnostic code. ICD-11 allows documentation of severity and functional impact, preserving diagnostic threshold while distinguishing clinical need. This precision has practical consequences for treatment planning, resource allocation, and outcome tracking.

Structural Reorganization in ICD-11

ICD-11 reorganizes mental and behavioral health classification based on updated understanding of how conditions relate to one another and what organizational structure best serves clinical utility across diverse settings. Reed and colleagues, describing the development process, articulated the guiding principles:

A primary goal of ICD-11 is for diagnostic guidelines to be usable by the full range of health professionals around the world who deliver mental health services, in contrast to the complexity of DSM-5 criteria. The clinical descriptions and diagnostic requirements are written in plain language, following principles of clinical utility, global applicability, and scientific validity. (Reed et al., 2019, p. 119)

The reorganization involved several structural changes. Neurodevelopmental disorders now appear at the beginning of the mental and behavioral health chapter, reflecting their typical onset early in life and their developmental trajectory. This placement supports a lifespan perspective that recognizes how conditions present differently at different ages.

Stress-related disorders are grouped together in a way that acknowledges their shared relationship to identifiable stressors. This grouping includes adjustment disorders, post-traumatic stress disorder, complex post-traumatic stress disorder, and prolonged grief disorder. Disorders due to substance use and addictive behaviors are organized to reflect current understanding of behavioral patterns that share features with substance-related conditions.

Table 8.1. Mental and Behavioral Health Classification Changes

DOMAIN	ICD-10 LIMITATION	ICD-11 IMPROVEMENT
Stress-related disorders	PTSD only; scattered placement across chapters	Coherent grouping; Complex PTSD added
Severity description	Minimal or absent; all cases treated as equivalent	Systematic within-diagnosis specifiers
Behavioral addictions	No recognition, conceptual gap	Gaming disorder included
Personality disorders	Fixed categorical types; poor reliability	Severity + trait domain model
Lifespan orientation	Childhood/adult diagnostic split	Unified lifespan framework

Note. ICD-11 addresses documented limitations in diagnostic reliability, cross-setting comparability, and clinical utility while maintaining meaningful diagnostic thresholds.

Dimensional Description and Severity

Perhaps the most significant conceptual shift in ICD-11's approach to mental and behavioral health is the increased emphasis on dimensional description. Rather than treating diagnostic categories as simply present or absent, ICD-11 provides tools for describing severity, specifying which features are present, and documenting functional impact.

Severity specifiers allow clinicians to indicate whether a condition is mild, moderate, or severe. This information has clinical relevance because severity affects treatment decisions, prognosis, and resource needs. It has research relevance because it enables investigators to characterize samples more precisely and to study how outcomes vary across the severity spectrum.

The dimensional approach does not imply reduced diagnostic rigor. Essential features remain specified for each condition. A patient must meet the required criteria to receive a diagnosis. What the dimensional approach adds is capacity to describe variation within diagnostic categories rather than treating all cases as equivalent once threshold is met.

Functional impact receives explicit attention in ICD-11's approach. The question is not merely whether symptoms are present but whether they impair the person's ability to function in important life domains. This emphasis aligns with broader trends in health classification that recognize disability and functioning as central to clinical significance.

Complex PTSD and Stress-Related Disorders

ICD-11 introduces Complex Post-Traumatic Stress Disorder as a distinct diagnosis, separate from but related to PTSD. This addition reflects accumulated clinical evidence that some patients exposed to prolonged or repeated trauma, particularly trauma of an interpersonal nature from which escape is difficult, develop a pattern of difficulties that extends beyond the core PTSD symptom profile.

The distinction between PTSD and Complex PTSD is not an expansion of diagnostic scope but a refinement of clinical description for presentations already widely recognized in practice. Complex PTSD includes the core PTSD features of re-experiencing, avoidance, and sense of current threat. It additionally includes disturbances in self-organization: difficulties with emotion regulation, negative self-concept, and disturbances in relationships.

The clinical utility of this distinction rests on its ability to identify patients whose treatment needs may differ from those with PTSD alone. Patients with difficulties in self-organization may require different therapeutic approaches or longer treatment courses. The classification does not prescribe specific treatments but provides vocabulary for identifying patients whose clinical picture includes these additional features.

Prolonged grief disorder, another addition in ICD-11, recognizes that some bereavement responses persist with an intensity and duration that constitutes a clinical disorder rather than normal grief. The broader reorganization of stress-related disorders creates a coherent grouping of conditions that share a relationship to identifiable stressors.

Personality Disorder Reclassification

ICD-11 introduces a fundamentally different approach to personality disorder classification. The shift to a severity-based model reflects evidence that impairment, not personality style, best predicts clinical need, prognosis, and resource utilization. Where ICD-10 specified categorical types such as borderline, antisocial, or narcissistic personality disorders, ICD-11 moves to a dimensional model based on severity and trait domains.

The new approach begins with an assessment of whether personality disorder is present and, if so, at what level of severity: mild, moderate, or severe. Severity is determined by the extent of disturbance in functioning across multiple domains including identity, self-direction, empathy, and capacity for closeness. This severity dimension provides clinically relevant information that the categorical approach obscured by treating all personality disorders as equivalent in seriousness.

Once severity is established, the classification provides five trait domains that can characterize the presentation: negative affectivity, detachment, dissociality, disinhibition, and anankastia. A patient may show prominent features in one domain, several domains, or present a pattern not well captured by any single domain. This approach accommodates the clinical reality that personality pathology does not sort neatly into discrete types.

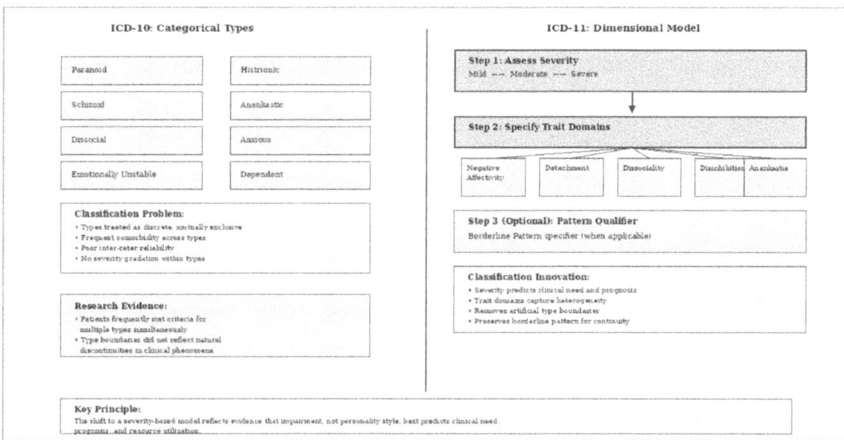

Figure 8.1. Personality Disorder Model. ICD-10's categorical types are replaced by a dimensional model assessing severity first, then characterizing trait domains. The borderline pattern specifier preserves continuity with prior research and clinical practice.

The reclassification addresses documented problems with the categorical approach. Research consistently showed that patients frequently met criteria for multiple personality disorder types simultaneously. Diagnostic reliability across clinicians was often poor. The boundaries between types did not appear to reflect natural discontinuities in the underlying phenomena.

One categorical specifier is retained: borderline pattern. This retention reflects both the extensive research literature using this designation and clinical familiarity with the presentation it describes. The borderline pattern qualifier can be applied when the clinical picture matches this well-recognized presentation, preserving continuity with prior research while embedding it within the broader dimensional framework.

What This Classification Does and Does Not Do

The scope of classification requires explicit delineation, particularly for mental and behavioral health where classification decisions carry substantial weight in clinical, social, and personal contexts.

The classification does provide recognized diagnostic categories based on current clinical consensus and available evidence. It does offer dimensional tools for describing severity and specifying features. It does reorganize conditions in ways intended to better reflect their relationships and to support clinical utility across diverse settings.

The classification does not define etiology. How mental and behavioral conditions arise, what relative contributions genetic, developmental, psychological, and social factors make, and how these factors interact are questions that classification cannot answer. The categories describe clinical presentations; they do not encode causal theories.

The classification does not prescribe treatment. Which interventions help which patients is determined by clinical research, not by how conditions are categorized. The classification does not replace clinical formulation. Diagnostic categories provide starting points for understanding individual patients; they do not substitute for comprehensive assessment.

The classification does not invalidate lived experience. How patients understand their own conditions, what meaning they make of their experiences, and what language they prefer are personal matters that classification does not govern.

Research and Health System Implications

The classificatory changes described in this chapter have implications for how research is conducted and how health systems organize mental and behavioral health services.

For research, the dimensional approach enables more precise characterization of study samples. Rather than treating all patients with a given diagnosis as equivalent, investigators can describe severity distributions and specify which features predominate. This precision supports both etiological research and treatment outcome studies by reducing heterogeneity within comparison groups.

For clinicians, the practical effect of these changes is improved documentation fidelity. Diagnoses can remain stable while severity and functional impact change over time. This supports continuity of care, reduces administrative churn, and produces cleaner longitudinal data for research and quality measurement. When documentation systems capture dimensional severity, health systems can distinguish populations requiring intensive intervention from those whose needs are less acute.

International comparability improves when the same classification is used across countries. Research findings become more generalizable. Epidemiological data become more interpretable. These benefits depend on consistent implementation, which remains a challenge when systems adopt new classifications at different rates.

Positioning for What Follows

Mental and behavioral health classification in ICD-11 reflects a broader shift occurring across the entire system: from rigid categories to clinically meaningful description, from static labels to dynamic understanding, and from fragmentation to coherence. The changes do not resolve every debate about mental illness, nor are they intended to. They provide a framework capable of evolving alongside clinical knowledge rather than constraining it.

The clinical domain chapters of this book have now examined chronic pain, neurodevelopmental conditions, post-viral syndromes, and mental and behavioral health. Each domain presented distinct classification challenges. Each required ICD-11 to develop approaches suited to the specific clinical phenomena involved. The common thread is classification adapting to clinical reality rather than forcing clinical reality into predetermined categories.

Chapter 9 integrates the implications of these clinical domain changes for research. How do the classification changes affect study design, cohort identification, and evidence synthesis? Chapter 10 addresses practical preparation for the transition, examining what infrastructure, training, and workflow changes are required to translate classificatory improvements into actual improvements in clinical documentation, research, and health system function.

PART III

RESEARCH AND SYSTEMS

9

RESEARCH AND DATA IMPLICATIONS

The preceding chapters examined how ICD-11 classifies specific clinical domains: chronic pain, neurodevelopmental conditions, post-viral syndromes, and mental and behavioral health. Each domain presented distinct classification challenges, and each required ICD-11 to develop approaches suited to the clinical phenomena involved. This chapter steps back from specific domains to address a question that applies across all of them: how does diagnostic classification shape what can be studied, counted, compared, and ultimately understood about health and disease? ICD-11 changes not only how conditions are coded, but what kinds of scientific questions can be asked, answered, and compared across populations.

This question matters because classification is not merely administrative. The codes that clinicians assign become the data that researchers analyze, that epidemiologists track, that health systems use for planning, and that policymakers cite when allocating resources. If the classification system cannot express clinically meaningful distinctions, those distinctions disappear from the data. If categories are unstable across settings or over time, comparisons become unreliable. If the system fragments related phenomena across incompatible codes, patterns that exist in clinical reality become invisible in research datasets.

Diagnosis as Research Infrastructure

Classification systems are easy to overlook. They operate in the background, shaping possibilities without calling attention to themselves. Bowker and Star, in their foundational analysis of classification and its consequences, captured this invisibility:

Classifications are powerful technologies. Embedded in working infrastructures they become relatively invisible without losing any of that power... Once a system is in place, the practical politics of these decisions are often forgotten. (Bowker & Star, 1999, pp. 319-320)

This observation applies directly to diagnostic classification. When a researcher queries a database for patients with a particular condition, the results depend entirely on how that condition was classified at the point of care. The classification determines who is counted and who is not, which cases can be compared and which cannot, whether a phenomenon appears in the data at all or remains invisible to systematic investigation.

The infrastructure metaphor is apt. Just as physical infrastructure enables or constrains what can be built upon it, classificatory infrastructure enables or constrains what can be known through health data. Research that draws on coded diagnostic data inherits whatever limitations exist in the classification system. A code added or removed, a boundary drawn or erased, a distinction preserved or collapsed—each of these choices reverberates through every study that subsequently uses the classification.

Limitations of ICD-10 for Contemporary Research

ICD-10 served research purposes for three decades. During that time, its limitations became increasingly apparent as research methods advanced and clinical understanding evolved. These limitations were not failures of the original design but consequences of a classification architecture developed before contemporary data science, electronic health records, and global health information exchange.

Fragmented coding across related phenomena created obstacles to cohort identification. Conditions now understood to share features were scattered across different chapters with incompatible coding logic. Exclusion hierarchies forced artificial choices that obscured clinical reality—when classification rules prohibited documenting co-occurring conditions, the resulting data reflected the rules rather than the patients.

Limited severity capture treated heterogeneous presentations as equivalent. A patient with mild impairment and a patient with severe disability might receive the same code, making them indistinguishable in research databases. Cross-study inconsistency undermined evidence synthesis: when different investigators used different coding approaches for the same clinical phenomena, meta-analysis became problematic and apparent disagreements might reflect coding differences rather than genuine clinical findings.

What ICD-11 Enables Scientifically

ICD-11's architectural redesign addresses these constraints. The changes are structural rather than merely additive, creating new possibilities rather than simply expanding the code set. Harrison and colleagues, reviewing ICD-11's information architecture, described the transformation:

ICD-11 was designed from the ground up using formal ontological principles, with each entity defined by its relationships to other entities in the system. This semantic structure supports automated reasoning, consistent application across contexts, and reuse of coded data for purposes beyond the original documentation. (Harrison et al., 2021, p. 8)

The Foundation's semantic structure means that relationships between entities are explicit and computable. Conditions that share features can be identified through their definitional properties, not just through manual cross-referencing. This enables research queries that would be impossible in a system where relationships exist only in human understanding.

Post-coordination enables documentation of clinical detail without requiring every possible combination to have its own pre-assigned code. Severity, laterality, temporal patterns, and other dimensions become available for analysis when documented through extension codes. Dimensional approaches within specific domains enable investigation of variation within diagnostic categories, supporting both etiological research and clinical trials.

The semantic structure of ICD-11 also enables emerging analytic approaches, including machine-assisted cohort identification and integration with AI-driven clinical decision support, in ways that legacy classifications could not support. The annual update cycle means that the classification can incorporate new knowledge without waiting for decadal revisions, reducing the lag between clinical understanding and classificatory representation.

Cohort Identification and Heterogeneity

Research quality depends substantially on how well study populations are defined. Cohorts that mix clinically distinct patients produce findings that may apply to none of them. ICD-11's expressive capacity supports more precise cohort definition across the clinical domains examined in earlier chapters.

Chronic pain research illustrates the challenge. Under ICD-10, patients with pain as their primary clinical problem were often coded by presumed etiology or affected body region, scattering them across the classification. ICD-11's dedicated chronic pain categories enable cohort identification based on the clinical problem itself, with post-coordination capturing mechanism, location, and severity.

Autism spectrum research encountered different obstacles. The categorical distinctions in ICD-10 created artificial boundaries that research increasingly could not justify. ICD-11's unified spectrum with dimensional specifiers enables cohorts defined by specific functional profiles rather than by categorical assignments that may have reflected diagnostic fashion as much as clinical reality.

Post-viral syndrome research requires tracking conditions whose manifestations are heterogeneous and whose boundaries with other conditions are contested. ICD-11's framework enables cohort identification based on explicit criteria, with post-coordination capturing specific symptom patterns and functional impacts. Complex PTSD research benefits from explicit recognition as distinct from PTSD, enabling research specifically on this population with clearer inclusion criteria.

Table 9.1. Research Capabilities: ICD-10 vs. ICD-11

RESEARCH TASK	ICD-10 LIMITATION	ICD-11 CAPABILITY
Severity stratification	Minimal or absent; cases treated as equivalent	Dimensional severity via extension codes
Co-occurrence documentation	Hierarchical exclusions forced single-diagnosis choice	Multiple conditions documentable without hierarchy
Longitudinal tracking	Code changes disrupted record continuity	Stable Foundation identifiers persist across updates
International comparison	National modifications diverged substantially	Common Foundation enables cross-national linkage
Cohort definition	Fragmented codes required ad hoc combinations	Unified concepts with post-coordination

Note: ICD-11's architectural features address infrastructural constraints that limited research capability under ICD-10, enabling more precise investigation across clinical domains.

Across all these domains, the common theme is reduction of artifactual heterogeneity. Clinical heterogeneity—genuine variation in how conditions present and progress—is scientifically interesting and clinically important. Artifactual heterogeneity—variation introduced by inconsistent classification—is noise that obscures signal. ICD-11's architecture reduces artifactual heterogeneity while preserving capacity to document and investigate clinical heterogeneity.

Longitudinal Tracking and Natural History

Many important research questions concern how conditions evolve over time. Do patients improve, stabilize, or worsen? What factors predict different trajectories? How do interventions affect long-term outcomes? Answering these questions requires tracking patients across encounters, often across years or decades.

ICD-10's revision history created discontinuities that complicated longitudinal research. Changes in category definitions, code assignments, and organizational structure meant that the same clinical presentation might receive different codes at different times, not because the patient changed but because the classification changed.

ICD-11's Foundation provides stable identifiers for clinical entities regardless of how they appear in specific linearizations. This stability means that changes in coding structure do not necessarily disrupt longitudinal tracking. An entity retains its identity in the Foundation even if its position in a linearization shifts. The dimensional approaches also support longitudinal research by enabling documentation of change within diagnostic categories—remission, recurrence, and fluctuation become documentable and therefore researchable.

International Comparability

Health research increasingly operates across national boundaries. Multi-site clinical trials, international epidemiological comparisons, and global disease surveillance all require that data from different countries can be meaningfully combined. Classification is the foundation of this comparability.

ICD-10's national modifications created substantial barriers to international comparison. ICD-10-CM in the United States, ICD-10-AM in Australia, and other national adaptations diverged not only in code specificity but sometimes in conceptual organization. Research findings from one country might not translate to another's coding system.

ICD-11's design explicitly prioritizes global applicability. The development process involved clinicians and researchers from diverse countries and health systems. The linearization model provides a mechanism for balancing global consistency with local adaptation. When research draws on Foundation-level identifiers rather than linearization-specific codes, international comparison becomes more feasible.

For policymakers and funding agencies, classification quality determines whether disease burden can be accurately estimated and whether interventions can be evaluated at scale. Conditions that cannot be reliably identified in administrative data remain invisible to cost-effectiveness analysis, workforce planning, and resource allocation. ICD-11's design reduces this invisibility by aligning diagnostic language with clinical reality rather than forcing clinical reality into legacy categories.

What This Does and Does Not Solve

Improved classification infrastructure creates possibilities. It does not guarantee that those possibilities will be realized, nor does it resolve the fundamental uncertainties that characterize medical knowledge. Clarity about what ICD-11 enables and what remains beyond its scope protects against both excessive skepticism and excessive optimism.

Misuse remains possible with any classification system; ICD-11 improves the tools available but does not control how they are used. Data can be selectively queried to support predetermined conclusions. Categories can be applied inconsistently despite clear definitions. Administrative and financial incentives can distort coding practice regardless of classification quality.

Better classification does not make classification equivalent to truth. Diagnostic categories remain human constructs, shaped by the knowledge and values of those who develop them. ICD-11 represents current consensus, which may evolve as understanding advances.

Better data infrastructure does not produce immediate answers. More precise cohort definition, more expressive documentation, and more consistent coding create conditions under which good research can occur. They do not substitute for the research itself. Uncertainty remains despite improved classification—many conditions have unknown etiology, contested boundaries, and unpredictable courses.

The realistic claim is that ICD-11 reduces certain obstacles to good research while creating new capabilities that ICD-10 could not provide. Whether these improvements translate into better clinical knowledge depends on how researchers, health systems, and institutions use the tools now available.

From Research Infrastructure to System Preparation

This chapter has traced the connections between diagnostic classification and research capability. The architectural features described in Chapter 4—the Foundation, linearizations, post-coordination, extension codes—have consequences for what can be studied and how reliably findings can be established. The clinical domain chapters, 5 through 8, each illustrated these consequences in specific contexts. This chapter drew those threads together into a general account of classification as research infrastructure.

The final chapters address a different kind of consequence: practical preparation. Health systems, clinical practices, and individual clinicians face concrete challenges in transitioning to ICD-11. Workflow changes, training needs, system modifications, and institutional adjustments all require attention. The improved capabilities described throughout this book remain theoretical until implementation makes them actual.

Chapter 10 provides guidance for that implementation. It addresses what organizations and individuals need to do, what timelines apply, what resources are available, and what pitfalls to avoid. The goal is to translate the conceptual understanding developed in preceding chapters into actionable preparation for a transition that, for many readers, lies in the near future.

10

THE U.S. CONTEXT

The preceding chapters have examined ICD-11's architecture, its clinical domain changes, and its implications for research and health data. This chapter turns to a different kind of question: why does ICD-11 adoption look different in different countries, and what specific factors shape the adoption process in the United States? The answer lies not in any single decision or policy but in the structural characteristics of how the U.S. health system is organized, governed, and financed.

Understanding the U.S. context matters for several reasons. Clinicians, researchers, and health system administrators working in the United States need to understand why ICD-11 implementation follows a different timeline than in other countries. International readers and organizations need to understand the institutional landscape that shapes U.S. health policy decisions. And anyone involved in preparing for eventual ICD-11 adoption needs to understand what that preparation involves given the particular features of the U.S. system.

This chapter provides that contextual understanding. It describes the governance structures, historical precedents, system characteristics, and regulatory processes that shape how the United States approaches classification transitions. The goal is explanation, not evaluation. Understanding how the system works is a prerequisite for any informed discussion of what should happen next. The United States' ICD-11 timeline is not an exception to global adoption patterns but an expression of the structural complexity of its healthcare governance.

ICD Adoption as a National Governance Process

The World Health Organization develops and maintains the International Classification of Diseases. It does not, however, mandate its adoption by member states. Each country retains sovereign authority over its health information systems, including decisions about which classification systems to use, when to adopt new versions, and how to adapt international standards to national contexts.

This governance structure means that WHO endorsement and national implementation are distinct processes. When WHO released ICD-11 in 2019 and member states endorsed it at the World Health Assembly, this established ICD-11 as the current international standard. It did not require any country to implement it by any particular date. Countries adopt ICD versions according to their own governance processes, institutional capacities, and policy priorities.

The United States participates actively in WHO classification development through the National Center for Health Statistics, which serves as the WHO Collaborating Centre for the Family of International Classifications. This participation reflects commitment to international standards and contributes U.S. clinical expertise to classification development. It does not, however, predetermine the timeline or process by which the U.S. implements new classification versions domestically.

Historical Precedent: ICD-9 to ICD-10 in the United States

The transition from ICD-9 to ICD-10 in the United States provides institutional memory that shapes current thinking about classification transitions. That experience, spanning more than two decades from initial planning to full implementation, illustrates both the complexity of classification changes in the U.S. context and the institutional capacity for eventually completing such transitions.

WHO released ICD-10 in 1990. The United States adopted ICD-10 for mortality coding relatively promptly, implementing it for death certificates in 1999. Morbidity coding, however, followed a different path. The development of ICD-10-CM, the clinical modification adapted for U.S. healthcare settings, required extensive work to preserve the clinical specificity that U.S. users had come to expect.

By implementation in 2015, ICD-10-CM contained more than 70,000 diagnosis codes, compared to approximately 14,000 in ICD-9-CM, reflecting the scale of system modification required. Electronic health record systems required modification. Billing and claims processing systems required reprogramming. Workforce training at scale required coordination across thousands of healthcare organizations. The compliance date, initially proposed for 2011, was ultimately implemented on October 1, 2015—a quarter century after WHO's release of ICD-10.

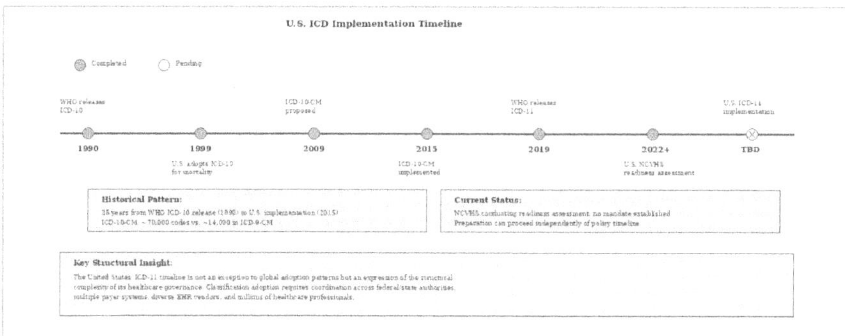

Figure 10.1. U.S. ICD Implementation Timeline. Historical pattern shows 25-year gap between WHO ICD-10 release and U.S. clinical implementation. Current ICD-11 adoption follows similar structural sequencing through NCVHS readiness assessment.

This history shapes current institutional thinking in several ways. Health system stakeholders remember the cost and disruption of the

ICD-10 transition. Policymakers recognize that implementation timelines must account for system-wide readiness, not just regulatory preference. The precedent does not dictate that ICD-11 adoption must follow a similar timeline, but it provides a realistic baseline for understanding what classification transitions involve in the U.S. context.

Fragmentation of the U.S. Health System

The United States does not have a unified national health system. Instead, it has multiple overlapping systems with different governance structures, financing mechanisms, and operational requirements. This fragmentation shapes how any system-wide change, including classification adoption, must be approached.

Payer diversity represents one dimension of fragmentation. Medicare, administered federally by the Centers for Medicare and Medicaid Services, covers elderly and disabled populations. Medicaid, jointly funded by federal and state governments but administered by states, covers low-income populations with substantial variation across state programs. Private insurers, ranging from large national carriers to regional plans, cover employed populations. Each payer system has its own claims processing infrastructure, coding requirements, and implementation timelines.

The electronic health record landscape reflects market-driven rather than centrally planned development. Multiple EHR vendors serve different segments of the healthcare market, each with their own development priorities and update cycles. A classification change requires that these vendors modify their systems, that healthcare organizations implement those modifications, and that the modifications work correctly across the interfaces that connect different systems.

Why the U.S. Is Not Canada

Comparisons to countries such as Canada, Australia, or the United Kingdom are common but often misleading. While these systems are decentralized in important respects, they retain national authority over core health information standards and payment mechanisms. In the United States, no single entity has comparable authority across payers, providers, and technology vendors. This distinction fundamentally alters what implementation requires.

Federal-state relationships add another layer of complexity unique to the U.S. context. Health policy authority is distributed across levels of government in ways that require coordination rather than command. States regulate insurance markets, license healthcare professionals, and administer Medicaid programs. Federal agencies set standards for Medicare and establish requirements that affect interstate commerce. Changes that require alignment across these levels involve negotiation and sequencing rather than unilateral implementation.

Regulatory Sequencing and Risk Management

Classification adoption in the United States proceeds through regulatory processes that involve multiple agencies, advisory bodies, and stakeholder input mechanisms. Understanding this sequencing clarifies why adoption timelines extend beyond what technical readiness alone might suggest.

The National Committee on Vital and Health Statistics serves as the statutory advisory body to the Secretary of Health and Human Services on health data and statistics matters, including classification systems. NCVHS does not set policy; it establishes the evidentiary and readiness foundation on which policy decisions are made. NCVHS has examined ICD-11 readiness through hearings, workgroups, and formal recommendations:

Any transition to a new code set requires careful assessment of the current state of readiness across the healthcare system, including the capacity of covered entities to implement changes, the availability of updated software and systems, the adequacy of training resources, and the potential for unintended consequences that could affect patient care or healthcare operations. (NCVHS, 2021)

The Centers for Medicare and Medicaid Services holds operational authority over the classification systems used for Medicare billing and, through its influence on industry standards, effectively shapes classification use across much of the U.S. healthcare system. Risk management considerations influence regulatory timing—a premature mandate could force implementation before systems are ready, potentially disrupting claims processing or affecting care documentation.

Table 10.1. Structural Factors Affecting ICD-11 Adoption in the United States

FACTOR	STRUCTURAL FEATURE	IMPLEMENTATION IMPLICATION
EHR ecosystem	Multiple vendors with independent development roadmaps	Vendor updates must precede provider adoption
Workforce scale	Millions of clinicians, coders, and billers	Training infrastructure must scale nationally
Federal-state structure	State-administered Medicaid; state licensing	Coordination across jurisdictions extends timelines
Payment linkage	Diagnosis codes tied to reimbursement	Risk of disruption requires staged rollout
Payer diversity	Medicare, Medicaid, commercial insurers	No single authority can mandate adoption

Note. These structural factors explain why U.S. adoption timelines differ from countries with centralized health information authority. Complexity requires coordinated sequencing, not resistance to change.

Parallel Use, Mapping, and Transitional Strategies

The path from current classification use to ICD-11 implementation need not involve an abrupt, system-wide switch. Various transitional strategies allow organizations to build familiarity with ICD-11 while maintaining operational continuity with current systems.

Parallel use involves working with ICD-11 for specific purposes while continuing to use ICD-10-CM for official reporting and billing. Research applications, clinical decision support development, and analytics projects can incorporate ICD-11 concepts without requiring changes to production billing systems.

For example, a health system might map ICD-11 chronic pain categories to existing ICD-10-CM codes for internal analytics and research, while continuing to submit claims using ICD-10-CM until a mandate is established. This approach allows organizations to develop expertise and identify implementation issues before facing compliance deadlines.

Mapping between classification systems enables translation of coded data across versions. WHO provides mapping tables between ICD-10 and ICD-11. Mapping is technically complex because the relationship between classification versions is not always one-to-one—some ICD-10 codes map to multiple ICD-11 options; some ICD-11 concepts have no direct ICD-10 equivalent. Mapping supports transition but does not eliminate the need for eventual native ICD-11 implementation.

What the U.S. Context Does and Does Not Imply

The structural factors described in this chapter shape the U.S. approach to ICD-11 adoption. They do not, however, support certain inferences that readers might be tempted to draw.

The current timeline does not imply rejection of ICD-11. The United States has not declined to adopt ICD-11 or expressed opposition to its content. The absence of an implementation mandate reflects the stage of the adoption process, not a negative judgment about the classification itself.

Caution about implementation timing does not imply ignorance of ICD-11's improvements. The clinical and structural advances described in earlier chapters are recognized by U.S. health informatics professionals, classification experts, and clinical specialists. Recognition of improvements and caution about implementation timing are not contradictory.

Complexity of the U.S. system does not imply resistance to change; it implies the need for coordinated sequencing. The same fragmented, multi-stakeholder system that complicates coordination also successfully completed the ICD-10 transition, implemented HIPAA transaction standards, adopted electronic prescribing, and made numerous other system-wide changes. Complexity requires more elaborate coordination mechanisms and longer timelines, but it does not preclude successful transitions.

The absence of a federal mandate does not imply absence of preparation. Healthcare organizations, EHR vendors, and professional associations can and do engage in preparation activities independent of regulatory requirements. Such preparation positions organizations for smoother transitions when mandates do arrive.

From Structural Context to Operational Readiness

This chapter has described the structural context that shapes

ICD-11 adoption in the United States. That context involves governance arrangements, historical precedents, system fragmentation, and regulatory processes that differ from those in many other countries. Understanding this context is necessary for realistic planning by anyone involved in U.S. healthcare classification use.

The concluding chapters address preparation from a practical standpoint. Given the structural context described here, what can organizations and individuals do to prepare for eventual ICD-11 implementation? What resources are available? What competencies require development? These questions concern readiness rather than advocacy—they address what to do given the situation as it exists, not arguments about what the situation should be.

The goal of preparation is to ensure that when implementation requirements are established, organizations and individuals are positioned to meet them effectively. The structural factors described in this chapter make clear that preparation cannot rely on short timelines or simple solutions. It requires sustained attention to building the knowledge, skills, and systems that ICD-11 implementation will demand.

PART IV

PREPARATION

11

PREPARING FOR TRANSITION

The preceding chapter described the structural context that shapes ICD-11 adoption in the United States. That context involves governance arrangements, historical precedents, and system characteristics that differ from those in many other countries. This chapter addresses a different question: given that context, what does preparation look like, and why does it matter even in the absence of implementation mandates? This chapter defines preparation as intellectual and organizational readiness, not operational execution.

Preparation, as discussed here, refers to building familiarity, developing understanding, and positioning for eventual transitions. It does not refer to operational implementation, system changes, or compliance activities. The distinction matters because preparation can proceed independently of policy timelines, creating value regardless of when mandates arrive. Understanding ICD-11's structure, recognizing its clinical implications, and developing literacy in its use are activities that benefit clinicians, researchers, and organizations whether implementation occurs in two years or ten.

This chapter describes what preparation involves across different domains: clinical understanding, research interpretation, education, and institutional awareness. The goal is to clarify what readiness means in this context and to explain why early engagement with ICD-11 concepts serves practical purposes even when no immediate action is required.

What Preparation Means in This Context

Preparation for a classification transition can mean different things in different contexts. Clarity about what this chapter means by preparation helps avoid misunderstanding about what is being suggested and what is not.

Preparation, as used here, does not mean implementation. Implementation involves operational changes: modifying billing systems, updating electronic health records, changing documentation workflows, retraining staff on new coding requirements. These activities occur in response to compliance deadlines and organizational decisions to adopt new systems.

Preparation also does not mean compliance. Compliance involves meeting regulatory requirements, following mandated standards, and ensuring that organizational practices align with external rules. In the current U.S. context, there are no ICD-11 compliance requirements for clinical documentation or billing.

Preparation, finally, does not mean advocacy. This chapter does not argue that clinicians or organizations should push for faster ICD-11 adoption, lobby for policy changes, or take positions on when transitions should occur.

What preparation does mean is knowledge acquisition and capacity building. It means developing familiarity with ICD-11's structure, understanding how it differs from ICD-10, recognizing its clinical implications, and building the conceptual foundation that makes eventual transitions smoother. This kind of preparation involves learning, not doing. In short, preparation is about knowing how the system works before being asked to use it.

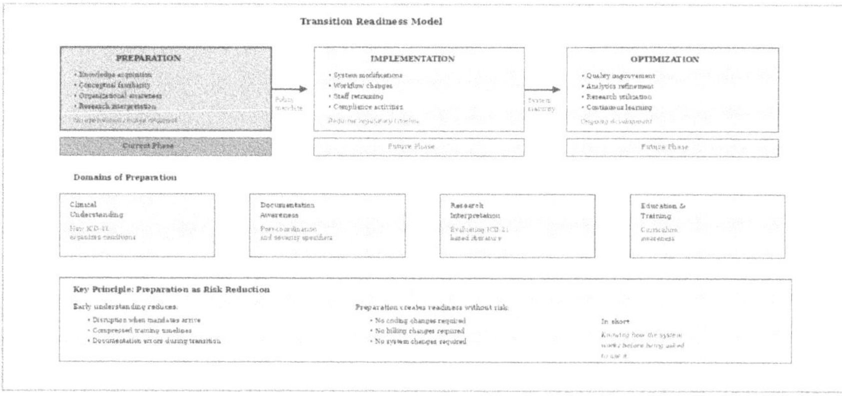

Figure 11.1. Transition Readiness Model. Preparation involves knowledge acquisition and conceptual familiarity without operational change. Implementation and optimization follow only after policy mandates are established.

Why Early Understanding Matters

Developing familiarity with ICD-11 before implementation requirements arrive serves several practical purposes. These benefits accrue regardless of adoption timelines and do not depend on any particular policy outcome.

Conceptual literacy reduces the learning burden when transitions do occur. Classification systems embody particular ways of organizing clinical information. ICD-11's dimensional approaches, post-coordination mechanisms, and reorganized clinical groupings reflect conceptual frameworks that differ from ICD-10's familiar structure. Clinicians and organizations that have already engaged with these concepts face a smaller adjustment when operational implementation begins.

Early understanding also supports interpretation of international research. As other countries implement ICD-11, published research increasingly uses ICD-11 categories and codes. Clinicians who understand how ICD-11 classifies conditions can better interpret findings from ICD-11-based studies and assess their applicability to U.S. practice.

WHO guidance on ICD-11 implementation acknowledges the value of phased engagement:

Countries may engage with ICD-11 at different levels depending on their circumstances and priorities. Familiarization with ICD-11 structure and content can proceed independently of decisions about official adoption timelines. Such early engagement supports informed planning and reduces implementation burden when transitions occur. (WHO, 2022)

Preparation as Risk Reduction

The phased approach that WHO describes recognizes that preparation and implementation are distinct activities that can proceed on different timelines. From an organizational perspective, early preparation functions as risk reduction.

Early understanding reduces disruption when mandates arrive. Organizations that have already familiarized staff with ICD-11 concepts face less compressed training timelines when compliance deadlines are established. Clinicians who understand dimensional approaches and post-coordination mechanisms require less intensive retraining than those encountering these concepts for the first time under deadline pressure.

Preparation also reduces documentation errors during transition periods. Classification transitions historically produce temporary increases in coding inconsistency as clinicians and coders learn new systems. Organizations with advance preparation experience shorter adjustment periods and fewer errors that require correction.

Domains of Preparation

Preparation for ICD-11 transition spans several domains, each involving different kinds of knowledge and different audiences. Understanding these domains helps clarify what preparation involves without implying that any particular activities are required.

Clinical understanding involves developing familiarity with how ICD-11 organizes clinical concepts. The clinical domain chapters of this book, covering chronic pain, neurodevelopmental conditions, post-viral syndromes, and mental and behavioral health, illustrated how ICD-11's approaches differ from ICD-10 in specific areas.

Documentation awareness involves recognizing how ICD-11's expressiveness affects what can be captured in coded data. The dimensional approaches, severity specifiers, and post-coordination mechanisms described in Chapter 4 enable more precise clinical description than ICD-10's categorical structure.

Research interpretation involves developing the ability to read and evaluate studies that use ICD-11 classifications. As the international research literature increasingly incorporates ICD-11, familiarity with its categories becomes important for evidence synthesis and clinical application.

Education and training involves considering how professional curricula might evolve to incorporate ICD-11 concepts. Educators developing training programs may benefit from understanding where ICD-11 introduces changes that warrant curricular attention.

Table 11.1. Domains of ICD-11 Preparation

DOMAIN	FOCUS	PURPOSE
Clinical understanding	How ICD-11 organizes conditions	Supports accurate interpretation and future documentation
Documentation awareness	Post-coordination and severity specifiers	Prepares clinicians for richer diagnostic description
Research interpretation	Reading ICD-11-based literature	Enables evaluation of international studies
Education and training	Curriculum awareness	Supports future workforce readiness

Note. None of these domains require operational change or compliance activity. Preparation involves learning and awareness, not system modification.

Institutional Readiness

Healthcare organizations can develop institutional readiness for ICD-11 transition without committing resources to implementation activities. Institutional readiness involves awareness, familiarity, and positioning rather than operational change.

Workforce familiarity develops when organizations provide opportunities for staff to learn about ICD-11. This might involve making educational resources available, supporting attendance at professional conferences that address ICD-11 topics, or facilitating internal discussions about classification changes.

Governance awareness involves ensuring that organizational leaders understand the classification landscape and its potential implications. Board members, executives, and clinical leaders benefit from understanding what ICD-11 represents and what eventual transitions might involve.

Vendor awareness involves understanding how electronic health record systems and other health information technologies might need to evolve to support ICD-11. Organizations can engage vendors in exploratory conversations about ICD-11 roadmaps without making procurement decisions.

Individual Clinician Preparation

Individual clinicians can develop ICD-11 familiarity through activities that align with ongoing professional development. These activities create value immediately while positioning clinicians for eventual transitions.

Understanding dimensional descriptions helps clinicians appreciate how ICD-11 approaches conditions that vary in severity, presentation, and functional impact. The shift from purely categorical classification to dimensional specification reflects evolving clinical understanding.

Interpreting post-coordinated diagnoses involves understanding how ICD-11 enables combination of stem codes with extension codes to create more precise clinical descriptions. Clinicians who understand this mechanism can better interpret ICD-11-coded data they encounter in research literature.

For example, a clinician reading an international study on chronic pain outcomes may encounter ICD-11 categories such as chronic primary pain or nociplastic mechanisms. Familiarity with these concepts allows accurate interpretation of findings even when domestic documentation systems still rely on ICD-10-CM. This interpretive capacity supports evidence-based practice regardless of domestic classification policy.

None of these activities require clinicians to change their current documentation or coding practices. They involve learning and reflection rather than operational change. Clinicians who engage with ICD-11 concepts do so as professional development, not compliance.

What Preparation Does and Does Not Require

Clarity about what preparation involves should extend to clarity about what it does not require. In the current U.S. context, preparation for ICD-11 transition involves no mandated changes to clinical or administrative practice.

No coding changes are required. Clinicians and coding professionals continue to use ICD-10-CM for all official documentation, billing, and reporting purposes. The classification system in use for U.S. healthcare operations remains ICD-10-CM until regulatory changes establish otherwise.

No billing changes are required. Healthcare organizations continue to submit claims using current code sets and billing processes. Nothing about ICD-11 preparation affects revenue cycle operations, payer interactions, or financial workflows.

No system changes are required. Electronic health records, practice management systems, and other health information technologies continue to operate with current classification support. System changes will occur when implementation requirements are established, not before.

No retraining mandate exists. Clinicians, coders, and other healthcare professionals are not required to complete ICD-11 training or demonstrate ICD-11 competency. Engagement with ICD-11 education is voluntary.

This clarity serves an important purpose: it reduces anxiety about whether preparation activities are somehow overdue or whether current practices are deficient. They are not. Preparation is an opportunity, not an obligation. Preparation creates readiness without risk; it does not place clinicians or organizations ahead of regulatory requirements.

Positioning for What Follows

This chapter has described what preparation for ICD-11 transition involves and why it matters even in the absence of implementation mandates. The emphasis has been on knowledge, familiarity, and readiness rather than operational change or compliance activity.

The final chapter of this book addresses a distinct set of considerations: billing, reimbursement, and administrative implications of classification transitions. Because classification interacts with payment systems in ways that introduce financial and regulatory risk, billing and reimbursement considerations warrant separate, cautious treatment.

Chapter 12 approaches these topics with the same descriptive orientation maintained throughout this book. It explains how classification and reimbursement interact, what kinds of questions arise during transitions, and what the historical record suggests about managing such transitions. It does not predict specific payment effects, recommend particular strategies, or advocate for policy positions. The goal, as throughout this book, is understanding rather than instruction.

12

BILLING AND DOCUMENTATION

Classification systems and payment systems interact in the U.S. healthcare environment in ways that create understandable confusion about what changes in one system imply for the other. This chapter addresses that confusion directly. Its purpose is to clarify what ICD-11 does and does not change with respect to billing, documentation, and administrative processes, providing the conceptual clarity that allows clinicians, administrators, and other stakeholders to engage with ICD-11 without misplaced anxiety. The intent is not to forecast change, but to clarify structure so that learning ICD-11 does not create unnecessary concern about obligations that do not yet exist.

The chapter does not provide billing instruction, coding guidance, or compliance strategies. Those topics require specificity that depends on policy decisions not yet made and regulatory requirements not yet established. What the chapter provides instead is demystification: an explanation of how classification and payment relate to each other, why they are distinct systems with different governance, and why changes in classification do not automatically or immediately translate into changes in billing practice.

This clarification matters because the ICD-10 transition left institutional memories that shape how healthcare stakeholders approach any classification change. That transition did involve billing changes, workflow disruptions, and significant organizational costs. Understanding why ICD-11 adoption, when it occurs, need not follow the same pattern requires understanding the structural relationships between the systems involved.

Why Administrative Questions Arise

Questions about billing and administrative implications arise naturally when healthcare professionals encounter discussions of ICD-11. This response reflects reasonable inference from experience, not confusion or ignorance. The inference, however, rests on assumptions about the relationship between classification and payment that warrant examination.

In the United States, ICD codes appear on virtually every healthcare claim. This ubiquity creates an association between diagnosis coding and payment that feels definitional. When clinicians think about ICD, they often think about billing. When administrators think about classification changes, they think about revenue cycle implications. These associations are not wrong—ICD codes do appear on claims and do affect payment—but they can obscure the distinction between the classification system itself and the payment systems that use it.

The ICD-10 transition reinforced these associations. That transition required extensive changes to billing systems, claims processing, and revenue cycle operations. Organizations invested substantial resources in system modifications, staff training, and workflow redesign. For many organizations, ICD-10 became synonymous with revenue risk, not because of the classification itself, but because classification and payment changes were tightly coupled in that transition. The experience was recent enough that institutional memory remains vivid. When ICD-11 is mentioned, the ICD-10 experience provides the reference frame.

Anxiety about billing implications is therefore understandable. It reflects learning from a consequential experience. What it does not reflect, however, is necessity. The relationship between classification adoption and billing change is contingent, not automatic. Understanding why requires examining how classification and payment systems actually relate to each other.

Separation of Classification and Payment

ICD is a classification system. It provides standardized vocabulary for describing diagnoses and health conditions. WHO develops and maintains ICD as a tool for mortality statistics, morbidity recording, and health information management. The classification itself is concerned with clinical description, not with payment determination.

Payment systems are payer-defined. Medicare, Medicaid, and private insurers establish their own rules for how diagnoses affect reimbursement. These rules reference ICD codes, but they are not determined by ICD. The classification provides the vocabulary; payers decide how to use that vocabulary in payment calculations. Different payers can and do use the same codes in different ways for payment purposes.

The National Committee on Vital and Health Statistics has consistently emphasized this distinction in its advisory communications regarding classification systems:

The adoption of a classification system for statistical and clinical purposes is distinct from its incorporation into payment methodologies. Classification provides standardized terminology for health information; payment policy decisions involve separate considerations including resource utilization, coverage determinations, and reimbursement rates that are established through regulatory and contractual processes independent of classification development. (NCVHS, 2022)

This distinction is foundational to U.S. health data governance and has been reaffirmed across multiple classification transitions. The separation means that ICD-11 adoption does not automatically trigger billing changes. A decision to use ICD-11 for mortality statistics, for example, would not affect claims processing. A decision to use ICD-11 in clinical documentation would not alter payment calculations until payers modified their systems to accept and process ICD-11 codes.

The practical implication is straightforward: classification change and billing change are not the same event. They can occur together, as they did in the ICD-10 transition, but they can also occur separately or in sequence. Understanding this separation reduces anxiety by clarifying that learning about ICD-11, understanding its structure, and even using it for certain purposes does not commit anyone to billing system changes.

Documentation Versus Coding

A related distinction separates documentation from coding. Documentation describes the clinical care provided to patients. Coding summarizes encounters using standardized categories for administrative purposes. These activities relate to each other but serve different functions and operate under different constraints.

Clinical documentation aims to capture the clinical picture accurately and completely. It supports continuity of care, clinical decision-making, and communication among providers. Good documentation describes what was observed, what was assessed, and what was done, with sufficient detail to support appropriate patient care. Documentation standards are established by professional norms, accreditation requirements, and institutional policies.

Coding translates documentation into standardized categories. Coders review clinical documentation and assign codes that represent the diagnoses and procedures documented. The codes then flow into administrative systems for billing, quality measurement, and other purposes. Coding accuracy depends on documentation quality, but coding requirements do not determine documentation requirements.

ICD-11's improved expressiveness, described in earlier chapters, enhances what classification can capture. Dimensional descriptions, post-coordination, and more precise categories enable coded data to represent clinical reality more accurately. However, improved classification capability does not create new documentation requirements. Clinicians continue to document according to existing standards. The classification's capability creates options; it does not create obligations.

Parallel Use, Mapping, and Transitional Tools

Classification transitions in complex health systems rarely occur as instantaneous switches. Various mechanisms support gradual transitions, allowing organizations to build familiarity with new systems while maintaining operational continuity with current ones.

Parallel use involves working with multiple classification systems simultaneously for different purposes. An organization might use ICD-11 for internal analytics or research while continuing to use ICD-10-CM for official reporting and billing. This approach allows exploration of ICD-11's capabilities without affecting production systems.

Mapping provides crosswalks between classification systems. WHO publishes mapping tables between ICD-10 and ICD-11, and national bodies develop additional mappings for clinical modifications. Mapping is inherently imperfect because classification systems are not simply different labels for identical concepts—some ICD-10 codes correspond to multiple ICD-11 options; some ICD-11 concepts have no direct ICD-10 equivalent.

These mechanisms exist to support transitions when they occur. They do not imply that transitions are imminent or that organizations should be actively implementing them. Understanding that such tools exist helps demystify how classification transitions work without suggesting that any particular organization needs to be using them now.

What ICD-11 Does Not Change

Clarity about what ICD-11 does not change is essential for reducing unnecessary concern. In the current U.S. context, ICD-11's existence does not alter established systems, requirements, or practices.

ICD-11 does not change current billing requirements. Healthcare organizations continue to submit claims using ICD-10-CM diagnosis codes. No payer currently requires or accepts ICD-11 codes for claims processing. Billing staff, revenue cycle operations, and claims processing workflows continue to operate with current code sets.

ICD-11 does not affect CPT codes. Current Procedural Terminology, maintained by the American Medical Association, provides procedure codes that are separate from diagnostic classification. CPT development follows its own processes independent of ICD version changes.

ICD-11 does not create payer mandates. Private insurers, Medicare, and Medicaid programs continue to operate under current coding requirements. No regulatory or contractual requirement compels payers to accept ICD-11 or providers to submit ICD-11 codes.

ICD-11 does not require electronic health record changes. EHR systems continue to support current classification systems. While vendors may develop ICD-11 capabilities in anticipation of future requirements, no current requirement obligates organizations to implement such capabilities.

ICD-11 does not create compliance obligations. No regulatory requirement mandates ICD-11 training, ICD-11 documentation, or ICD-11 system readiness. Organizations are not deficient, behind, or at risk because they have not implemented ICD-11.

Table 12.1. What ICD-11 Changes and What It Does Not

DOMAIN	ICD-11 IMPACT	CURRENT STATUS
Billing	None	All claims continue under ICD-10-CM
CPT Procedure Codes	None	CPT maintained independently
Documentation Standards	None	Professional and accreditation standards unchanged
Payer Policies	None	No payer mandates ICD-11
EHR Requirements	None	No required system changes
Compliance	None	No ICD-11 obligations exist

Note. This table reflects the current U.S. regulatory environment. Future policy decisions may establish requirements not yet in effect.

Institutional Risk Management

Healthcare organizations appropriately manage risk by avoiding premature commitment to changes that are not yet required. This caution reflects sound institutional governance, not resistance to improvement or failure to prepare.

Classification transitions involve costs. System modifications, staff training, workflow changes, and productivity effects during transition periods all require resources. Organizations reasonably defer these costs until requirements are clear and timelines are established. Premature investment risks wasted resources if requirements change or timelines extend.

Staged evaluation protects organizations from implementation problems. Waiting to observe early adopters' experiences, learning from implementation challenges encountered elsewhere, and allowing systems to mature before organizational adoption all reduce risk. Organizations that adopt after initial implementation issues have been identified and addressed face fewer disruptions than early adopters.

Caution also protects against unintended consequences. Classification changes can have effects that are difficult to anticipate, particularly in complex systems with many interdependencies. In large healthcare systems, delayed adoption is often a marker of governance discipline rather than resistance to innovation. This risk management perspective explains why organizations may be cautious about ICD-11 even while recognizing its improvements. The question is not whether ICD-11 offers benefits but whether the timing is right for organizational investment in transition.

Closing Perspective

This chapter completes the main text of the book. The chapters have traced a path from the foundations of diagnostic classification through ICD-11's architecture, clinical domain changes, research implications, the U.S. context, and practical considerations for preparation and administration. Throughout, the orientation has been explanatory rather than prescriptive, aiming to build understanding rather than direct action.

The appendices that follow provide reference materials that support this understanding. Crosswalk summaries illustrate relationships between ICD-10 and ICD-11 categories in selected clinical domains. A glossary defines technical terms used throughout the book. A resource guide points to official sources for those seeking additional information. These materials are informational, not prescriptive.

The book's goal has been to provide the conceptual foundation that allows healthcare professionals, researchers, administrators, and policymakers to engage with ICD-11 knowledgeably. That engagement may take different forms for different readers: clinical understanding, research interpretation, institutional planning, or policy analysis. Whatever form it takes, informed engagement serves better than either anxious avoidance or premature action. Informed engagement allows systems to change deliberately rather than reactively, and deliberation is the hallmark of durable healthcare reform.

BIBLIOGRAPHY

American Health Information Management Association. (2015). ICD-10-CM/PCS transition: Planning and preparation. Author.

American Psychiatric Association. (2022). Diagnostic and statistical manual of mental disorders (5th ed., text rev.). Author.

Ashar, Y. K., Gordon, A., Schubiner, H., Uipi, C., Knight, K., Anderson, Z., Carlisle, J., Poliber, L., Geuter, S., Flood, T. F., Kragel, P. A., Dimidjian, S., Lumley, M. A., & Wager, T. D. (2022). Effect of pain reprocessing therapy vs placebo and usual care for patients with chronic back pain: A randomized clinical trial. *JAMA Internal Medicine, 182(1), 64–73*. https://doi.org/10.1001/jamainternmed.2021.6669

Bach, B., & First, M. B. (2018). Application of the ICD-11 classification of personality disorders. *BMC Psychiatry, 18(1)*, Article 351. https://doi.org/10.1186/s12888-018-1908-3

Baliki, M. N., Petre, B., Torbey, S., Herrmann, K. M., Huang, L., Schnitzer, T. J., Fields, H. L., & Apkarian, A. V. (2012). Corticostriatal functional connectivity predicts transition to chronic back pain. *Nature Neuroscience, 15(8), 1117–1119*. https://doi.org/10.1038/nn.3153

Benoliel, R., Svensson, P., Evers, S., Wang, S.-J., Barke, A., Korwisi, B., Rief, W., & Treede, R.-D. (2019). The IASP classification of chronic pain for ICD-11: Chronic secondary headache or orofacial pain. *Pain, 160(1), 60–68*. https://doi.org/10.1097/j.pain.0000000000001435

Bennett, M. I., Kaasa, S., Barke, A., Korwisi, B., Rief, W., & Treede, R.-D. (2019). The IASP classification of chronic pain for ICD-11: Chronic cancer-related pain. *Pain, 160(1), 38–44*. https://doi.org/10.1097/j.pain.0000000000001363

Bertillon, J. (1903). Nomenclature des maladies: Statistique de morbidité, statistique des causes de décès. Imprimerie typographique de l'école d'Alembert.

Bodenreider, O. (2004). The Unified Medical Language System (UMLS): Integrating biomedical terminology. *Nucleic Acids Research, 32(Database issue)*, D267–D270. https://doi.org/10.1093/nar/gkh061

Bowker, G. C., & Star, S. L. (1999). Sorting things out: Classification and its consequences. MIT Press.

Brewin, C. R. (2020). Complex post-traumatic stress disorder: A new diagnosis in ICD-11. *BJPsych Advances, 26(3), 145–152*. https://doi.org/10.1192/bja.2019.48

Brewin, C. R., Cloitre, M., Hyland, P., Shevlin, M., Maercker, A., Bryant, R. A., Humayun, A., Jones, L. M., Kagee, A., Rousseau, C., Somasundaram, D., Suzuki, Y., Wessely, S., van Ommeren, M., & Reed, G. M. (2017). A review of current evidence regarding the ICD-11 proposals for diagnosing PTSD and complex PTSD. *Clinical Psychology Review, 58, 1–15*. https://doi.org/10.1016/j.cpr.2017.09.001

Centers for Disease Control and Prevention. (2022). CDC clinical practice guideline for prescribing opioids for pain. *MMWR Recommendations and Reports, 71(3), 1–95.* https://doi.org/10.15585/mmwr.rr7103a1

Centers for Medicare and Medicaid Services. (2024). ICD-10-CM official guidelines for coding and reporting. Author.

Cimino, J. J. (1998). Desiderata for controlled medical vocabularies in the twenty-first century. *Methods of Information in Medicine, 37(4–5), 394–403.*

Clark, L. A., Cuthbert, B., Lewis-Fernández, R., Narrow, W. E., & Reed, G. M. (2017). Three approaches to understanding and classifying mental disorder: ICD-11, DSM-5, and the National Institute of Mental Health's Research Domain Criteria (RDoC). *Psychological Science in the Public Interest, 18(2), 72–145.* https://doi.org/10.1177/1529100617727266

Fagot-Largeault, A. (2006). The roots of the International Classification of Diseases. *Medical History, 50(1), 117–124.*

Farr, W. (1839). First annual report of the Registrar-General of births, deaths, and marriages in England. Her Majesty's Stationery Office.

Feinstein, A. R. (1967). Clinical judgment. Williams & Wilkins.

Fitzcharles, M.-A., Cohen, S. P., Clauw, D. J., Littlejohn, G., Usui, C., & Häuser, W. (2021). Nociplastic pain: Towards an understanding of prevalent pain conditions. *The Lancet, 397(10289), 2098–2110.* https://doi.org/10.1016/S0140-6736(21)00392-5

GBD 2019 Diseases and Injuries Collaborators. (2020). *Global burden of 369 diseases and injuries in 204 countries and territories, 1990–2019.* The Lancet, 396(10258), 1204–1222. https://doi.org/10.1016/S0140-6736(20)30925-9

GBD 2021 Low Back Pain Collaborators. (2023). *Global, regional, and national burden of low back pain, 1990–2020.* The Lancet Rheumatology, 5(6), e316–e329. https://doi.org/10.1016/S2665-9913(23)00098-X

Greaves-Lord, K., Skuse, D., & Mandy, W. (2022). Innovations of the ICD-11 in the field of autism spectrum disorder. *Clinical Psychology in Europe, 4(Suppl.)*, Article e10005. https://doi.org/10.32872/cpe.10005

Harrison, J. E., Weber, S., Jakob, R., & Chute, C. G. (2021). ICD-11: An international classification of diseases for the twenty-first century. *BMC Medical Informatics and Decision Making, 21(Suppl. 6)*, Article 206. https://doi.org/10.1186/s12911-021-01534-6

Institute of Medicine. (2011). Relieving pain in America: A blueprint for transforming prevention, care, education, and research. National Academies Press.

Institute of Medicine. (2015). Beyond myalgic encephalomyelitis/chronic fatigue syndrome: Redefining an illness. National Academies Press.

International Association for the Study of Pain. (2017). IASP terminology. https://www.iasp-pain.org/resources/terminology/

Jakob, R., & Dee, R. (2021). *ICD-11 implementation or not? Bulletin of the World Health Organization, 99(3), 203–204.* https://doi.org/10.2471/BLT.20.278234

Jensen, M. C., Brant-Zawadzki, M. N., Obuchowski, N., Modic, M. T., Malkasian, D., & Ross, J. S. (1994). Magnetic resonance imaging of the lumbar spine in people without back pain. *The New England Journal of Medicine, 331(2), 69–73.* https://doi.org/10.1056/NEJM199407143310201

Jetté, N., Quan, H., Hemmelgarn, B., Drosler, S., Maass, C., Moskal, L., Paoin, W.,

Sundararajan, V., Gao, S., Jakob, R., Ustun, B., & Ghali, W. A. (2010). The development, evolution, and modifications of ICD-10. *Medical Care, 48(12), 1105–1110*. https://doi.org/10.1097/MLR.0b013e3181ef9d3e

Jutel, A. (2011). Putting a name to it: Diagnosis in contemporary society. Johns Hopkins University Press.

Keeley, J. W., Reed, G. M., Roberts, M. C., Evans, S. C., Medina-Mora, M. E., Robles, R., Rebello, T., Sharan, P., Gureje, O., First, M. B., Andrews, H. F., Ayuso-Mateos, J. L., Gaebel, W., Zielasek, J., & Saxena, S. (2016). Disorders specifically associated with stress. *International Journal of Clinical and Health Psychology, 16(2), 109–127*. https://doi.org/10.1016/j.ijchp.2015.09.002

Komaroff, A. L., & Bateman, L. (2021). *Will COVID-19 lead to ME/CFS? Frontiers in Medicine, 7*, Article 606824. https://doi.org/10.3389/fmed.2020.606824

Kosek, E., Clauw, D., Nijs, J., Baron, R., Gilron, I., Harris, R. E., Mico, J.-A., Rice, A. S. C., & Sterling, M. (2021). Chronic nociplastic pain. *Pain, 162(11), 2629–2634*. https://doi.org/10.1097/j.pain.0000000000002324

Kotov, R., Krueger, R. F., Watson, D., Achenbach, T. M., Althoff, R. R., Bagby, R. M., Brown, T. A., Carpenter, W. T., Caspi, A., Clark, L. A., Eaton, N. R., Forbes, M. K., Forbush, K. T., Goldberg, D., Hasin, D., Hyman, S. E., Ivanova, M. Y., Lynam, D. R., Markon, K., . . . Zimmerman, M. (2017). The Hierarchical Taxonomy of Psychopathology (HiTOP). *Journal of Abnormal Psychology, 126(4), 454–477*. https://doi.org/10.1037/abn0000258

Krueger, R. F., Hobbs, K. A., Conway, C. C., Dick, D. M., Dretsch, M. N., Eaton, N. R., Forbes, M. K., Forbush, K. T., Keyes, K. M., Latzman, R. D., Michelini, G., Patrick, C. J., Sellbom, M., Slade, T., South, S. C., Sunderland, M., Tackett, J. L., Waldman, I., Waszczuk, M. A., . . . HiTOP Utility Workgroup. (2021). Validity and utility of Hierarchical Taxonomy of Psychopathology (HiTOP): II. Externalizing superspectrum. *World Psychiatry, 20(2), 171–193*. https://doi.org/10.1002/wps.20844

Lord, C., Elsabbagh, M., Baird, G., & Veenstra-Vanderweele, J. (2018). Autism spectrum disorder. *The Lancet, 392(10146), 508–520*. https://doi.org/10.1016/S0140-6736(18)31129-2

Maercker, A., Brewin, C. R., Bryant, R. A., Cloitre, M., van Ommeren, M., Jones, L. M., Humayan, A., Kagee, A., Llosa, A. E., Rousseau, C., Somasundaram, D. J., Souza, R., Suzuki, Y., Weissbecker, I., Wessely, S. C., First, M. B., & Reed, G. M. (2013). Diagnosis and classification of disorders specifically associated with stress: Proposals for ICD-11. *World Psychiatry, 12(3), 198–206*. https://doi.org/10.1002/wps.20057

Madden, R. H., & Musgrove, P. (2020). The ICD-11 era. *International Journal of Environmental Research and Public Health, 17(16)*, Article 5926. https://doi.org/10.3390/ijerph17165926

Moriyama, I. M., Loy, R. M., & Robb-Smith, A. H. T. (2011). History of the statistical classification of diseases and causes of death. National Center for Health Statistics.

Nalbandian, A., Sehgal, K., Gupta, A., Madhavan, M. V., McGroder, C., Stevens, J. S., Cook, J. R., Nordvig, A. S., Shalev, D., Sehrawat, T. S., Ahluwalia, N., Bikdeli, B., Dietz, D., Der-Nigoghossian, C., Liyanage-Don, N., Rosner, G. F., Bernstein, E. J.,

Mohan, S., Beckley, A. A., . . . Wan, E. Y. (2021). Post-acute COVID-19 syndrome. *Nature Medicine, 27(4), 601–615.* https://doi.org/10.1038/s41591-021-01283-z

National Center for Health Statistics. (2024). ICD-10-CM. Author.

National Committee on Vital and Health Statistics. (2003). Report to the Secretary of HHS on ICD-10. Author.

National Committee on Vital and Health Statistics. (2021). ICD-11 and U.S. morbidity classification: Recommendations. Author.

National Committee on Vital and Health Statistics. (2022). Letter to the Secretary of HHS regarding ICD-11 planning. Author.

Nightingale, F. (1859). Notes on hospitals. John W. Parker and Son.

Reed, G. M., First, M. B., Kogan, C. S., Hyman, S. E., Gureje, O., Gaebel, W., Maj, M., Stein, D. J., Maercker, A., Tyrer, P., Claudino, A., Garralda, E., Salvador-Carulla, L., Ray, R., Saunders, J. B., Dua, T., Poznyak, V., Medina-Mora, M. E., Pike, K. M., . . . Saxena, S. (2019). Innovations and changes in the ICD-11 classification of mental, behavioural and neurodevelopmental disorders. *World Psychiatry, 18(1), 3–19.* https://doi.org/10.1002/wps.20611

Rodrigues, J. M., Robinson, D., Della Mea, V., Campbell, J., Rector, A., Schulz, S., Brear, H., Üstün, B., Spackman, K., Millar, J., Chute, C. G., & Jakob, R. (2015). Semantic alignment between ICD-11 and SNOMED CT. *Studies in Health Technology and Informatics, 216, 790–794.* https://doi.org/10.3233/978-1-61499-564-7-790

Rosenberg, C. E., & Golden, J. (Eds.). (1992). Framing disease. Rutgers University Press.

Schug, S. A., Lavand'homme, P., Barke, A., Korwisi, B., Rief, W., Treede, R.-D., & IASP Taskforce for the Classification of Chronic Pain. (2019). The IASP classification of chronic pain for ICD-11: Chronic postsurgical and posttraumatic pain. *Pain, 160(1), 45–52.* https://doi.org/10.1097/j.pain.0000000000001413

Smith, B. H., Fors, E. A., Korwisi, B., Barke, A., Cameron, P., Colvin, L., Richardson, C., Rief, W., Treede, R.-D., & IASP Taskforce for the Classification of Chronic Pain. (2019). The IASP classification of chronic pain for ICD-11: Applicability in primary care. *Pain, 160(1), 83–87.* https://doi.org/10.1097/j.pain.0000000000001360

Soriano, J. B., Murthy, S., Marshall, J. C., Relan, P., & Diaz, J. V. (2022). A clinical case definition of post-COVID-19 condition. *The Lancet Infectious Diseases, 22(4)*, e102–e107. https://doi.org/10.1016/S1473-3099(21)00703-9

Stein, D. J., Szatmari, P., Gaebel, W., Berk, M., Vieta, E., Maj, M., de Vries, Y. A., Roest, A. M., de Jonge, P., Maercker, A., Brewin, C. R., Pike, K. M., Grilo, C. M., Fineberg, N. A., Briken, P., Cohen-Kettenis, P. T., & Reed, G. M. (2020). Mental, behavioral and neurodevelopmental disorders in the ICD-11: An international perspective on key changes and controversies. *BMC Medicine, 18(1)*, Article 21. https://doi.org/10.1186/s12916-020-1495-2

Tebartz van Elst, L., Riedel, A., & Biscaldi-Schäfer, M. (2025). Reclassification of neurodevelopmental disorders in ICD-11. *Der Nervenarzt, 96(Suppl. 1)*, 40–47. https://doi.org/10.1007/s00115-022-01379-4

Topaz, M., Shafran-Topaz, L., & Bowles, K. H. (2013). ICD-9 to ICD-10. *Perspectives in Health Information Management, 10(Spring), 1*d.

Treede, R.-D., Rief, W., Barke, A., Aziz, Q., Bennett, M. I., Benoliel, R., Cohen, M., Evers,

S., Finnerup, N. B., First, M. B., Giamberardino, M. A., Kaasa, S., Kosek, E., Lavand'homme, P., Nicholas, M., Perrot, S., Scholz, J., Schug, S., Smith, B. H., . . . Wang, S.-J. (2015). A classification of chronic pain for ICD-11. *Pain, 156(6), 1003*–1007. https://doi.org/10.1097/j.pain.0000000000000160

Treede, R.-D., Rief, W., Barke, A., Aziz, Q., Bennett, M. I., Benoliel, R., Cohen, M., Evers, S., Finnerup, N. B., First, M. B., Giamberardino, M. A., Kaasa, S., Korwisi, B., Kosek, E., Lavand'homme, P., Nicholas, M., Perrot, S., Scholz, J., Schug, S., . . . Wang, S.-J. (2019). Chronic pain as a symptom or a disease: The IASP Classification of Chronic Pain for the International Classification of Diseases (ICD-11). *Pain, 160(1), 19*–27. https://doi.org/10.1097/j.pain.0000000000001384

Tyrer, P., Reed, G. M., & Crawford, M. J. (2015). Classification, assessment, prevalence, and effect of personality disorder. *The Lancet, 385(9969), 717*–726. https://doi.org/10.1016/S0140-6736(14)61995-4

U.S. Department of Health and Human Services. (2023). Report to Congress on health IT progress. Office of the National Coordinator.

Vos, T., Flaxman, A. D., Naghavi, M., Lozano, R., Michaud, C., Ezzati, M., Shibuya, K., Salomon, J. A., Abdalla, S., Aboyans, V., Abraham, J., Ackerman, I., Aggarwal, R., Ahn, S. Y., Ali, M. K., Alvarado, M., Anderson, H. R., Anderson, L. M., Andrews, K. G., . . . Murray, C. J. L. (2012). Years lived with disability (YLDs) for 1160 sequelae of 289 diseases and injuries 1990–2010: A systematic analysis for the Global Burden of Disease Study 2010. *The Lancet, 380(9859), 2163*–2196. https://doi.org/10.1016/S0140-6736(12)61729-2

World Health Organization. (2001). International Classification of Functioning, Disability and Health. Author.

World Health Organization. (2007). History of the development of the ICD. https://www.who.int/standards/classifications/classification-of-diseases/history-of-icd

World Health Organization. (2019a). International statistical classification of diseases and related health problems (11th rev.). Author.

World Health Organization. (2019b). ICD-11 implementation or adaptation guide. Author.

World Health Organization. (2019c). Seventy-second World Health Assembly resolution WHA72.15: ICD-11. Author.

World Health Organization. (2020). Maintaining and updating the ICD: The ICD update and revision process. Author.

World Health Organization. (2022a). ICD-11 for mortality and morbidity statistics (MMS). https://icd.who.int/browse/2024-01/mms/en

World Health Organization. (2022b). ICD-11 reference guide. https://icd.who.int/icd11refguide/en/index.html

World Health Organization. (2022c). ICD-11 training tool. https://icd.who.int/training/

World Health Organization. (2023). Transition to ICD-11: Guidance for countries. Author.

World Health Organization. (n.d.). ICD-11 implementation: Frequently asked questions. https://www.who.int/standards/classifications/frequently-asked-questions/icd-11-implementation

APPENDIX A

GLOSSARY OF ICD-11 TERMINOLOGY

Core Classification Terms

Cluster Coding

Combining multiple ICD-11 codes to represent complex clinical scenarios with appropriate specificity.

Extension Code

A code beginning with 'X' that adds specificity (severity, anatomy, etiology) when combined with a stem code. Cannot be used alone.

Foundation

The comprehensive semantic network containing all ICD-11 entities, definitions, and relationships from which linearizations derive.

ICD-11 MMS

ICD-11 for Mortality and Morbidity Statistics—the primary linearization for clinical coding and health statistics.

Linearization

A hierarchical subset of the Foundation organized for specific purposes (mortality, morbidity, primary care).

Multiple Parenting

Structural feature allowing entities to appear under multiple parent categories, reflecting clinical reality.

Post-Coordination

Combining codes at time of use to create precise diagnostic expressions beyond single-code specificity.

Pre-Coordination

Multiple concepts built into a single code, as in ICD-10-CM. ICD-11 reduces reliance on this approach.

Sanctioning Rules

ICD-11 rules specifying which extension codes can legally attach to which stem codes, preventing invalid combinations.

Stem Code

A code usable independently to represent a health condition; foundation of diagnostic expressions.

URI (Uniform Resource Identifier)

Unique, permanent identifier for each ICD-11 entity in the Foundation, enabling precise reference across systems and time.

WHO-FIC

World Health Organization Family of International Classifications including ICD-11, ICF, and ICHI.

Chronic Pain Terms

Chronic Primary Pain

Pain persisting >3 months that is the primary clinical problem, not explained by another condition (e.g., fibromyalgia).

Chronic Secondary Pain

Pain persisting >3 months arising from identifiable underlying condition (cancer, surgery, neuropathy).

Nociplastic Pain

Pain from altered nociception without clear tissue damage or nerve lesion—explains conditions where traditional models fail.

Neurodevelopmental Terms

Autism Spectrum Disorder

Consolidated ICD-11 category replacing autism, Asperger's, and PDD-NOS with dimensional specifiers.

Dimensional Specifiers

Codes describing variation within a diagnosis (intellectual functioning, language capacity for ASD).

Mental Health Terms

Bodily Distress Disorder

ICD-11 category replacing somatoform disorders; characterized by distressing bodily symptoms and excessive attention to them.

Complex PTSD

PTSD plus self-organization disturbances: affect dysregulation, negative self-concept, interpersonal difficulties.

Dimensional Model

ICD-11's personality disorder approach: severity levels + trait domains replacing categorical types.

Gaming Disorder

Impaired control over gaming with functional impairment for 12+ months.

Prolonged Grief Disorder

Grief persisting beyond expected duration causing significant functional impairment.

APPENDIX B

QUICK REFERENCE BY CLINICAL DOMAIN

Chronic Pain

Chronic Pain: ICD-10 vs. ICD-11

ICD-10 APPROACH	ICD-11 APPROACH
Pain by anatomical location	Pain by mechanism and pattern
No unified pain framework	Dedicated chronic pain chapter
Structural OR psychological	Primary/secondary distinction
Severity not systematic	Extension codes for severity

Chronic Primary Pain (MG30.0): Pain is the primary problem

MG30.00 Widespread • MG30.01 Musculoskeletal • MG30.02 Visceral • MG30.03 Headache

Chronic Secondary Pain (MG30.1-6): Pain from underlying condition

Cancer • Postsurgical • Musculoskeletal • Visceral • Neuropathic • Headache

Severity: XS7T Mild • XS2G Moderate • XS4C Severe

Autism Spectrum Disorder (6A02)

Autism Spectrum Disorder (6A02): ICD-10 vs. ICD-11

ICD-10	ICD-11
Multiple diagnoses	Single spectrum
Childhood focus	Lifespan orientation
Categorical subtypes	Dimensional specifiers

Required specifiers:

Intellectual: 6A02.0 Without / 6A02.1 With disorder of intellectual development

Language: .x0 Mild/none / .x1 Impaired / .x2 Absent

Severity: XS7T Mild • XS2G Moderate • XS4C Severe

Post-Viral Syndromes

RA02 Post COVID-19 condition: Symptoms 3+ months after SARS-CoV-2

8E49 Postviral fatigue syndrome: Chronic fatigue after documented viral infection

8E49.0 ME/CFS: When ME/CFS criteria met

Mental Health

Personality Disorders: Severity (Mild/Moderate/Severe) + Trait domains

Traits: Negative Affectivity • Detachment • Dissociality • Disinhibition • Anankastia

Trauma: 6B40 PTSD • 6B41 Complex PTSD • 6B42 Prolonged grief

New: 6C51 Gaming disorder • Bodily distress disorder

APPENDIX C

IMPLEMENTATION READINESS CHECKLIST

For Clinicians

☐ Understand primary/secondary distinction in your clinical domains

☐ Learn post-coordination concept and basic extension codes

☐ Review key code changes in your specialty

☐ Complete ICD-11 training module (free at WHO)

☐ Practice using ICD-11 browser (icd.who.int)

☐ Document severity and functional impact systematically

☐ Create quick reference for your high-volume diagnoses

☐ Identify patients whose diagnoses will change significantly under ICD-11

For Practice Managers

☐ Inventory current ICD-10 utilization patterns

☐ Identify high-volume codes with significant ICD-11 changes

☐ Assess EHR vendor ICD-11 readiness and timeline

☐ Evaluate coding staff training needs

☐ Budget for training and productivity impacts

☐ Establish ICD-11 working group

☐ Develop communication plan for clinical staff

For Health Systems

☐ Confirm EHR ICD-11 capability and upgrade schedule
☐ Test ICD-11 code entry in staging environment
☐ Validate claim submission pathways with payers
☐ Update documentation templates for ICD-11 specificity
☐ Schedule comprehensive coding staff training
☐ Define coding accuracy metrics for monitoring
☐ Plan pre/post transition audit process
☐ Coordinate with NCVHS updates on federal timeline recommendations

APPENDIX D

DOCUMENTATION TEMPLATES

Note: These templates are conceptual frameworks for adaptation to specific EHR platforms.

D.1 Chronic Pain Assessment

Location: ______ Duration: ______ Quality: □ Aching □ Burning □ Stabbing □ Other

Intensity (0-10): Rest ___ Average ___ Worst ___

Classification: □ Chronic Primary Pain □ Chronic Secondary Pain

If Primary: □ Widespread □ Musculoskeletal □ Visceral □ Headache

If Secondary: Underlying condition: ______ Type: □ Cancer □ Postsurgical □ Neuropathic

Pain mechanism: □ Nociceptive □ Neuropathic □ Nociplastic □ Mixed

Severity: □ Mild □ Moderate □ Severe Functional impact: ______

D.2 Neurodevelopmental Evaluation

Social Communication: □ Reciprocity deficits □ Nonverbal deficits □ Relationship deficits

Restricted Patterns: □ Stereotyped □ Sameness □ Restricted interests □ Sensory

Intellectual: □ Without disorder (6A02.0) □ With disorder (6A02.1)

Language: □ Mild/none (.x0) □ Impaired (.x1) □ Absent (.x2)

Severity: □ Mild □ Moderate □ Severe Support needs: ______

D.3 Post-Viral Documentation

Triggering infection: □ COVID-19 □ EBV □ Other □ Unknown Onset: ______

Duration since acute infection: ______ months

Symptoms: □ Fatigue □ PEM □ Cognitive □ Autonomic □ Respiratory □ Pain

Function: Work __% baseline Physical __% baseline ADLs __% baseline

Trajectory: □ Improving □ Stable □ Fluctuating □ Worsening

D.4 Mental Health (Dimensional)

Depression: □ None □ Mild □ Moderate □ Severe Anxiety: □ None □ Mild □ Moderate □ Severe

Trauma: □ Single □ Prolonged Core PTSD: □ Re-experiencing □ Avoidance □ Hyperarousal

Complex PTSD: □ Affect dysreg □ Negative self □ Interpersonal difficulties

Personality: Severity □ Mild □ Mod □ Severe Traits: □ NegAff □ Det □ Diss □ Disin □ Anan

Functional impact: □ Occupational □ Social □ Self-care GAF equivalent: __

D.5 Prolonged Grief Assessment

Loss: Relationship to deceased: ______ Date of death: ______

Duration since loss: ______ months (6+ months required for adults)

Core symptoms: □ Intense longing/yearning □ Preoccupation with deceased

Associated: □ Disbelief □ Avoidance □ Difficulty moving on □ Numbness □ Identity disruption

Functional impairment: □ Occupational □ Social □ Self-care Severity: □ Mild □ Mod □ Severe

APPENDIX E

RESOURCES FOR CONTINUED LEARNING

WHO Resources

ICD-11 Browser: icd.who.int — Official interface for exploring codes and definitions

Coding Tool: icd.who.int/ct11 — Build diagnostic expressions with post-coordination

Training: who.int/standards/classifications/training — Free educational modules

Reference Guide: icd.who.int/icd11refguide — Comprehensive documentation

U.S. Federal Resources

CMS: cms.gov — Federal agency for ICD implementation timelines and Medicare policy

NCHS: cdc.gov/nchs — Will develop ICD-11-CM when transition authorized

NCVHS: ncvhs.hhs.gov — Federal advisory body recommending ICD-11 adoption timelines

Professional Organizations

IASP: iasp-pain.org — Developed chronic pain classification; educational materials

AHIMA: ahima.org — Primary U.S. source for ICD-11 implementation guidance

AHA: aha.org — Publishes Coding Clinic, official ICD coding guidance

Integral Neuroscience Initiative

Website: integralneuroscience.org — U.S. ICD-11 implementation resources and updates

Resource Library: Updated links and materials maintained as federal guidance evolves

Key Publications

Reed et al. (2019). Innovations in ICD-11 mental disorders. World Psychiatry, 18(1).

Treede et al. (2019). IASP Chronic Pain Classification for ICD-11. Pain, 160(1).

Harrison et al. (2021). ICD-11: An international classification for the twenty-first century. BMC Medical Informatics, 21(Suppl. 6).

First et al. (2021). Comparison of ICD-11 and DSM-5. World Psychiatry, 20(1).

Key Search Terms for Staying Current

ICD-11 implementation • ICD-11-CM development • NCVHS ICD-11 recommendations • CMS ICD transition • ICD-11 MMS updates • Post-coordination coding • ICD-11 clinical utility

APPENDIX F

ICD-11 CHANGES ACROSS MEDICAL SPECIALTIES

This book examines four clinical domains in depth: chronic pain, neurodevelopmental conditions, post-viral syndromes, and mental health. ICD-11's changes extend across virtually every medical specialty. This appendix provides a high-level overview to help readers understand what colleagues in other fields are facing and how referral relationships may be affected.

Palliative Care & Hospice

Palliative Care & Hospice

KEY CHANGES	CLINICAL IMPACT
Chronic pain integration	MG30 codes capture pain as primary problem in end-of-life care
Dimensional severity	Extension codes document declining function over time
Symptom clustering	Post-coordination captures multi-symptom reality (fatigue + pain + dyspnea)
Prolonged grief (6B42)	New code supports hospice bereavement services documentation
Functioning assessment	ICF-linked codes support hospice eligibility documentation

Note: ICD-11's dimensional approach aligns with Total Pain philosophy

—physical, psychological, social dimensions documented through post-coordination rather than single diagnosis.

Integrative & Complementary Medicine

Integrative & Complementary Medicine

KEY CHANGES	CLINICAL IMPACT
Chapter 26: Traditional Medicine	New optional chapter for acupuncture, TCM, and traditional medicine diagnoses
Pattern diagnoses	TCM concepts (Qi stagnation, Cold-dampness) now have standardized codes
Dual coding	WHO recommends TM codes alongside Western diagnoses, not instead of
Adverse event tracking	Codes for harm from complementary therapies (PL01, PK81.3) enable safety monitoring

Note: Chapter 26 is optional—countries choose whether to implement. U.S. adoption status is undetermined, but integrative practitioners should be aware of its existence.

Cardiology

Cardiology

KEY CHANGES	CLINICAL IMPACT
Sleep-wake disorders chapter	Sleep apnea/cardiac risk documentation improved; organic/non-organic distinction removed
Hypertensive disease refinement	More precise classification of hypertensive heart and kidney disease
Stroke reclassification	Now classified as neurological disorder; affects cardiology/neurology coordination
Post-coordination	Laterality, severity, and anatomical detail through extension codes

Oncology

Oncology

KEY CHANGES	CLINICAL IMPACT
Restructured neoplasm chapter	Complete reorganization of cancer classification structure
Behavior as extension codes	Benign/malignant/uncertain behavior now coded via extensions, not separate codes
Staging documentation	Post-coordination enables more precise staging and grading documentation
Cancer-related pain	Chronic secondary cancer pain (MG30.1) provides dedicated pain coding

Neurology

Neurology

KEY CHANGES	CLINICAL IMPACT
Headache alignment	Headache disorders aligned with ICHD-3 international classification
Dementia restructuring	Dementia classification reorganized; behavioral specifiers improved
Stroke reclassification	Now in neurology chapter rather than circulatory; refined subtypes
Chronic neuropathic pain	MG30.5 provides specific coding for chronic neuropathic pain conditions

Infectious Disease

Infectious Disease

KEY CHANGES	CLINICAL IMPACT
COVID-19 codes	RA01 (confirmed), RA02 (post-COVID) integrated into classification
Antimicrobial resistance	New codes for documenting resistant organisms
Emerging pathogens	Annual update cycle allows rapid addition of new infectious agents
Post-viral syndromes	8E49 postviral fatigue and ME/CFS now explicitly codable

Rheumatology

Rheumatology

KEY CHANGES	CLINICAL IMPACT
Chronic pain overlap	Chronic musculoskeletal pain codes intersect with rheumatologic conditions
Fibromyalgia recognition	MG30.01 chronic widespread pain captures fibromyalgia as primary pain condition
Autoimmune reorganization	Systemic autoimmune conditions reorganized with improved specificity
Severity documentation	Dimensional severity approach applicable to chronic rheumatologic conditions

Endocrinology

Endocrinology

KEY CHANGES	CLINICAL IMPACT
Diabetes refinement	More precise staging and complication documentation
Metabolic conditions	Improved recognition of metabolic syndrome components
Thyroid reorganization	Thyroid disorders restructured with clearer classification logic

Pediatrics

Pediatrics

KEY CHANGES	CLINICAL IMPACT
Developmental specifiers	Developmental period specifiers available throughout classification
Neurodevelopmental changes	ASD, ADHD, and learning disorders restructured (see Chapter 6)
Feeding/eating disorders	ARFID and other pediatric-relevant eating conditions reorganized
Perinatal coding	Improved perinatal condition coding with gestational timing specifiers

Emergency Medicine

Emergency Medicine

KEY CHANGES	CLINICAL IMPACT
External cause restructuring	External cause codes reorganized for clearer injury documentation
Injury coding	Streamlined injury coding with mechanism and intent specifiers
Poisoning/toxicity	Substance-related harm codes improved for ED documentation

Primary Care

Primary Care

KEY CHANGES	CLINICAL IMPACT
Primary care linearization	Dedicated ICD-11 Primary Care subset available for high-volume settings
Simplified coding option	Less complex coding for common conditions in resource-limited settings
Chronic disease management	Severity documentation supports chronic care coordination
Mental health integration	Clearer mental health codes support integrated behavioral health models

This overview is not exhaustive. Every medical specialty will encounter ICD-11 changes relevant to their practice. The common thread across all specialties is the shift from rigid categorical coding to flexible, dimensional documentation that better captures clinical reality. Clinicians are encouraged to explore ICD-11 codes specific to their specialty using the WHO browser at icd.who.int.

ABOUT THE AUTHORS

ELIZABETH TEKLINSKI, PhD, LPC, NCC, NPT-C

Founder & President

Dr. Teklinski's career began in hospice and palliative care, where she trained in Dame Cicely Saunders' Total Pain philosophy recognizing physical, psychological, emotional, social, and spiritual dimensions of suffering. Her background spans chronic pain intervention, clinical operations, and neuropsychotherapy.

She is EMDR Institute-trained and completed coursework through NICABM in neuroscience, trauma therapy, and mental health. She trained in Pain Reprocessing Therapy, the approach producing 66% pain-free outcomes in a 2021 JAMA study.

She holds a PhD in East-West Psychology from CIIS and is a Licensed Professional Counselor. In 2019, she received a Special Tribute from the State of Michigan for leadership in passage of House Bill 4325. She serves on the MMHCA Board and provides monthly Medicare Q&A sessions for counselors statewide.

MICHELLE O'CONNOR-TEKLINSKI, LMSW

Co-Founder & Chief Program Officer

Michelle O'Connor-Teklinski has spent more than thirty years working with neurodivergent individuals and their families. She has held executive positions at NEXT for AUTISM, Hope Network, Judson Center, and MI-UCP. At Hope Network, she developed a partnership with Michigan State University's College of Human Medicine for autism diagnosis and research.

ICD-11 reflects the inclusive approach Michelle has championed throughout her career. She holds an MSW from Wayne State University and is a graduate of the National Leadership Institute on Developmental Disabilities.

ANDREW TEKLINSKI, MD, MS, FACC, CCDS, RPVI

Co-Founder & Chief Medical Officer

Dr. Teklinski is board-certified in Internal Medicine and Cardiovascular Disease, a Fellow of the American College of Cardiology, and holds certifications as a Clinical Cardiac Device Specialist and Registered Physician in Vascular Interpretation.

His research portfolio includes more than twenty major clinical outcome trials. He has served as Principal Investigator on multiple Phase III trials, and his work has shaped treatment guidelines used by physicians worldwide.

ABOUT THE INTEGRAL NEUROSCIENCE INITIATIVE

Building the Diagnostic Infrastructure America Needs

The Integral Neuroscience Initiative was founded to address a fundamental gap in American healthcare: a diagnostic system decades behind modern science.

ICD-11, the World Health Organization's updated classification, has been in effect globally since 2022. It enables diagnostic accuracy that outdated codes cannot provide. INI was founded when clinicians, researchers, and systems leaders recognized that no U.S. infrastructure existed to bring ICD-11 into clinical practice.

We exist to help American patients access what the rest of the world already has. We operate independently, without commercial, payer, or vendor influence.

What We Build

ICD-11 provides the diagnostic architecture modern medicine needs. Codes alone don't change practice. We build what clinicians and health systems need: training programs, curriculum resources, diagnostic decision support, crosswalks, billing guidance, readiness assessments, and policy translation.

Our Unique Role

INI is the only organization in the United States focused exclusively on ICD-11 operationalization. What's missing is the implementation infrastructure that turns a new classification into changed clinical practice. INI fills that gap.

Organization

The Integral Neuroscience Initiative is a 501(c)(3) public charity registered in Michigan. We are noncommercial and independent. Our work is funded entirely through foundation grants and individual contributions.

EIN: 85-0630961

CONNECT WITH INI

Partner With Us

Health systems, professional associations, EHR vendors, and educational institutions preparing for ICD-11 can work with INI on training, implementation planning, and curriculum development.

Support Our Work

As a 501(c)(3) public charity, INI relies on foundation grants and individual contributions. Your tax-deductible donation supports the development of free implementation resources for clinicians nationwide.

Stay Informed

Visit integralneuroscience.org for updates on U.S. ICD-11 implementation timelines, new resources, and training opportunities.

Contact

info@integralneuroscience.org

integralneuroscience.org

Donate

integralneuroscience.org/donate

Diagnosis shapes treatment. Treatment shapes outcomes.
Better diagnosis is where better medicine begins.

www.ingramcontent.com/pod-product-compliance
Lightning Source LLC
LaVergne TN
LVHW050934210926
848482LV00013B/611
* 9 7 9 8 9 9 4 2 5 8 1 2 5 *